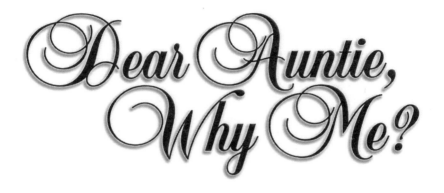

Dear Auntie, Why Me?

A Duluth Woman's Breast Cancer Story

By "Peggy" Margaret A. Anderson

Front Cover by Mary Boman | Book Illustrations by Joel Skinner

First Edition

Published and Printed by: Pro Print 326 E. Central Entrance Duluth, MN 55811 U.S.A

Distributed by: Peggy Anderson Publishing 5204 Otsego St. Duluth, MN 55804
1-800-900-4559-00(pin) maande1@charter.net

This book is not intended to be a substitute for professional medical advice. You,
the reader should always consult with your doctor before embarking on any change of
treatment.

The information I have provided is what I, as the author, feel is correct and reliable.

This book is dedicated to the following SMDC staff: Dr. David Frye (Miller Dwan Radiation), Dr. Eric Hoyer (Duluth Clinic Radiation), Dr. James Krook (Duluth Clinic Oncology), Roma Myers (Duluth Clinic Sonograhy), Miller Dwan Radiation Staff, Dr. Ingrid Nisswandt (Lakeside Medical Center), Dr. Audrey Park Skinner (Duluth Clinic Surgery), and Lisa Starr MSN, C-NP (Duluth Clinic Breast Program Coordinator).

The following individuals are recognized for their exceptional knowledge and skills in diagnosing and treating breast cancer: Dr. David Frye who helped me through the radiation process by answering my numerous questions with his caring ways, Dr. Eric Hoyer who diagnosed my breast cancer immediately, Dr. James Krook guided me with through hard treatment choices with his sense of humor. Roma Myers who identified my breast cancer by her thorough ways. Miller Dwan Radiation staff helped me through the radiation process by way of compassion and a sense of humor. Dr. Ingrid Nisswandt who has always treated my health throughout the years with dedicated thoroughness. Dr. Park Skinner, who was the surgeon that skillfully performed three surgeries on me. Lisa Starr, an extremely knowledgeable nurse practitioner, who helped my husband and I to understand the cancer diagnosis, and go through the difficult process with her positive encouragement.

The proceeds from this book will be donated to the SMDC Foundation in honor of the above named individuals. Proceeds will provide support for Breast Cancer Center diagnostic and treatment equipment and for Breast Cancer Center staff training and development.

I would like to dedicate this book to the following family members: Jim Anderson, who was by my side each step of the process. I also want to dedicate this book to my aunt, Karen McDonald, who lived through this ordeal day by day with me. Both have given me enormous amount of love and support to complete this book project by editing, reading it over and over. I also want to thank my children, Chris and Lisa, for being there when I needed them.

This book is dedicated to Dr. James Krook and his wife, Mary, who both have had cancer and survived.

The cover of this book is dedicated to the illustrator, Mary Boman (married to Dr. Tom Boman, UMD), who lost her daughter, Annette Boman to cancer. Annette was a UMD professor and cancer researcher.

Finally, I would like to dedicate my writing to all who have bought this book to learn more about breast cancer and how it can be prevented. It is dedicated to those who have lost a friend, family member, acquaintance or helped someone through the cancer process. It is dedicated to all survivors as well.

Acknowledgements

I am grateful to the following family members for their support: Sharen Lapham, Lynn Mackin, Jim McDonald, Kay and Dick Studley.

In particular, I want to thank the following friends and organizations for their support, stories, and kind words of encouragement: Sue and Tom Bernard, Wendy Braun, Nancy Brown, Central Staff, Colleen Dougherty, Linda Duhaime, Duluth Police Reserves, Linda Eastman, Pam Egbert, Carolyn Graves, Jaima and Tom Hanson (Embers),Russ Herring, Frank Hoder, Deb Jarvis, Pastor Joe Koranda, Margie and Ward Lane, Eric Lassila, Sharon and Jerry Lassila, Lester Park Citizens Patrol, Donna Lundahl, Gwen Lundberg, Elaine and Jim McMann, Ward Melenich, Members of Faith Lutheran Church, Tricia Neubarth, Helen Rivers, Diane Schmitz, Bob Schulz, Ruth Wittmers, Millie and Jake Zollar.

I want to mention the excellent care from doctors and staff at the Duluth Clinic, Miller Dwan and St. Mary's Medical Center: Cynthia Anderson (Allergy Dept.), Diane Bierke-Nelson (Genetics Dept.), Dr. Stephen Bloom (Gynecology), Lois Korkow (PT Lakeside), Kim Lakhen (Otolaryngology), Dr. Wade Lillegard (Orthopedics), Dr. David McNaney (Radiation), Diane Nelson (Oncology),Julie Rollin (Patient Relations), Dr. Daniel Skorich (Ophthalmology), SMDC Foundation, Dr. Theresa Smith (Gastroenterology), St. Mary's Surgery, Dr. Christine Swenson (Hermantown Duluth Clinic), Miller Dwan/Duluth Clinic Breast Support Group, Miller Dwan Foundation, Miller Dwan Surgery, Dr. Rolofo Urias (Radiation).

In our community, I want to recognize help from the following individuals and organizations: Heidi's Mastectomy Shop, Linda Pugliese and Toby Sillanpa (Duluth American Cancer), Pete Reynolds (Gold Cross), Kim Storm (YWCA Breast Awareness Program), Dr. Dean Weber (Northland Plastic and Reconstructive Surgery), and Walgreens Plaza Pharmacy.

At the district and national level, I want to recognize the help I have received from: Karla Gomez (Blue Cross-Blue Shield of Minnesota case manager), Life Extension Advisors, National American Cancer Society, National Cancer Institute, Janice Rannow (Minnesota American Cancer Society), and SEER/National Statistics.

Also, I want to acknowledge the stories and experiences shared with me about cancer by so many individuals in the community. This is for those individuals who have known someone with breast cancer or who have died from this disease. This book does not list every one but a few that I want to mention.

Central High School Memorial Recognition
Sue Bodin whose husband was Ralph Bodin, my former assistant principal, died of metastic breast cancer. Also Katherine Anderson former Central High School teacher.

This book is a series of letters written to my Auntie about my breast cancer diagnosis, search for answers, and treatment. In some cases I have included her reply to my letters. There are medical facts, terminology, knowledge, concepts, pictures, and charts, so that she could be informed and have the information in written and visual forms. We have exchanged positive affirmations, thoughts, and information about our daily lives as well.

With this life changing diagnosis, I searched high and low to find answers to many questions. I needed to do this, so that I could understand why this happened, understand the choice of treatments and how I could prevent a reoccurrence. My aunt and doctor felt it would be therapeutic experience for me to write this book. In doing so I read magazines, newspaper and internet articles, library books, watched videos, bought books, and read books in the radiation library at Miller Dwan. A lot of information was received from medical personnel as well. I wanted my daughter and my cousins to know about breast cancer and to inform other women. This must be the teacher in me. If breast cancer information was easier to find, maybe more women would stay informed, and try to prevent this disease.

Many questions still remain for me. Was there some way I could have prevented this from happening? Then the question I had for myself was, "What could I do to change this?" In education classes we always learned there is a cause and effect. There are always pre tests and post tests to see if the material was learned. I see the same in breast cancer treatment. There are diagnostic tests, treatments, and follow up tests. If we survey patients to see what they have been doing, looking for patterns as possible causes, we may be able to treat them by a holistic approach in the attempt to save more lives. I didn't want to be just a statistic like some of the women with metastatic breast cancer that I heard about in the community.

This is a letter that I received from my Auntie on 11/5/04.

Dear Peggy,

I am so proud that you are writing a book to share your personal experience with breast cancer. The good and the bad, the ups and downs, the scary moments and great people you met along your way of seeking treatment for breast cancer.

As you remember, at the start of your problem--a lump, unread mammogram, and questionable test results, I encouraged you to always request a copy of all of your test results to start a file for yourself. This way you could keep track of what's been done, when it was done, and question any results that you didn't understand. You followed through by checking things on the internet, doing a lot of reading, and researching.

Your efforts put you in a position to be your own best advocate for your health. When consulting specialists you knew what they were talking about. You knew what questions you needed answers to. You knew what information was needed to make a decision for your choice of treatments.

As your cancer file expanded and your personal experiences with breast cancer increased, we discussed your desire to put this information in some form for your daughter and my daughters. This desire led to your decision to write this book, so that you could share your experience with anyone facing breast cancer.

My hope is that through sharing what you have learned and what you have experienced, that you will give encouragement to all women facing breast cancer to help them find the answers to their questions in their battle with breast cancer.

Love always,

Aunt Karen

Contents

"I have no special gift. I am only passionately curious."   -Albert Einstein

4/30/04

Dear Auntie Karen,

   Today amidst the sharp cold front I am sitting here wondering if Duluth, the San Francisco of the North, looks any different than a year ago. Soon the weather will transmute and people will see the true signs of spring emerge. I just can't wait to see the vivid celebrations as the trees start budding and the birds chirping. The dirty brown snow left by winter will dissipate from the swimming pool and hot tub cover. This year we won't be able to start our pool up right way. Dave Twining Electrical Company needs to install a new electrical service in our outside garage as the pool's service needs to be brought up to code. The old power system under the chain link fence as you recall was sparking this winter. Our hot tub was used only once this winter. The changing of the seasons seems to control our everyday lives and choices.

   I hope this letter finds you well. You said the other night you had a lot of intense spring cleaning and grocery shopping to do. Please don't over do it.

   This afternoon I had an appointment with Dr. Nisswandt, my family physician. This appointment was made because I felt a one inch hard lump in my left breast. You know, some people "do this touchy feely breast self exam" with their breasts each month, but not me. I felt a lump in 2001. If you recall I had a mammogram, ultrasound and biopsy at that time. These procedures are not foreign to me. Religiously, I do go for a mammogram each year because I do know from reading books, magazines and the internet that finding tumors at an early state is often curable. I also know that mammograms are the best standard of care for most women. At some point of time in our lives we can get lumps, and they are not always cancerous. There's a risk with having having mammograms over and over, but we don't have a lot of other diagnostic tools to detect breast tumors at this time. The chance of early detection outweighs the risk of breast cancer. My doctor could also feel this lump, so she referred me for an ultrasound, mammogram and to see a surgeon. She is thinking it will take a long time to get in to see the surgeon.

When was the last time you had a mammogram? I was so surprised to hear that you have never done a self exam of your breast. The American Cancer Society tells people in their literature that there's a 1 in 7 chance that women will develop invasive breast cancer in their life time. The mammogram is the first step in diagnosing cancer. So it is very important that we do these screening exams and look for the signs. I am enclosing a diagram showing you how it is done from the American Cancer Society.

Furthermore, you must schedule your mammogram each year. Breast Cancer is the 2nd leading cause of death in women. It's a disease that can be prevented if caught early. Breast cancer increases with age. A mammogram can pick up calcium deposits, slow moving tumors, and early DCIS (ductual cancer in situ). If you get tubular and irregular calcium deposits these are often cancerous. All suspicious lumps need to have a biopsy even though eighty percent are benign. It is important to have an early diagnosis of breast cancer because it will save your life and increase your treatment options.

I had an ultrasound on 2/28/01 and a biopsy on 3/9/01 of my left breast. The ultrasound report stated it was the right breast and when it really was the left breast. At times I had a lot of breast pain, and discharge from my nipple. I dread the compression on my very dense breasts. My doctor once suggested to take a pain pill before having this procedure done. I later got a report on this breast, as you suggested I get copies of all my reports. The initial report stated there were "findings that were highly suspicious for malignancy," BIRAD 3 . After the steterotactic biopsy the report read, "fibrocystic changes with some focal calcifications." There was no mention of a blood vessel that broke or my breast would turn black later. Instead theradiology report stated "no immediate complications." The biopsy pathological and surgical report showed I had " benign breast tissue samples with fibrocystic changes." It also stated there was "focal mild ductual hyperplasia" and microcalcification deposits associated with benign lobule and vessels present." Remember I had this procedure in 2001 because I read later on The National Cancer Institute web site that atypical hyperplasia puts you at risk for breast cancer. I wondered about this and the scar tissue that seemed to be developing in my breast. Six months later I had another ultrasound and mammogram and passed with flying colors. What we women go through!

A little flashback about the biopsy in 2001. I don't know if you recall this but the surgical tape broke off too soon, and I had to go to have it re-taped at Lakeside Medical Center. By that time I had a black breast. I had joked with a fellow colleague at Central High School, Russ, that this year I'd be sending out multicultural Christmas cards. When he asked me, "Why?" I said, "I have one white breast and one black from a blood vessel breaking during my biopsy." Russ said he was anxious to get one of my Christmas cards!

Oh, I'm starting to think about people who have died of breast cancer. This is because I read the *Daily Guideposts* you gave me and wrote in. I read that my great grandmother, Karen Meier died in 1942 at age 79 of metastatic breast cancer and pneumonia. Then I started thinking about my paternal grandmother, Edna Meier Prahl, dying in 1955 of metastatic breast cancer after being diagnosed in 1936. She lived a long time after this poor diagnosis. It got me thinking about who else on my Father's side of the family may have had breast cancer. Years ago I did a family member medical tree of diseases relatives had died from but not breast cancer. What can you tell me about my Father's side of the family?

I thought you'd like the explanation of how to do a breast self exam, some breast diagrams, facts, terminology, knowledge and concepts that are becoming a part of my new vocabulary.

Lovingly,

Peggy, your niece

Symptoms of Breast Cancer, Benign Findings,
Diagnostic Tests, Reports
Cancer Facts, Terms, Knowledge, Concepts

Symptoms of Breast Cancer:
There's a change in the breast or nipple:
-tenderness, pain, burning, the breast may feel irritated (These are not considered a sign of early breast cancer.)
-lump or change in size of the breast
-thickening in the breast, near the breast, under the arms or in the lymph node areas
-the veins in the breast could be changed
-the nipple could be dimpled, retracted or inverted inward
-the nipple could be red, be scale like, pitted, ulcerated, or it could have ridges
-the nipple could have a spontaneous fluid discharge that is clear or bloody

Who should have a mammogram? The American Cancer Society states in their 1999 pamphlet women age 40 and over should have annual mammograms, annual clinical breast exams by a trained doctor or nurse and do monthly breast self-exams. At ages 20-39 women should have a clinical breast exam by a trained doctor or nurse every three years, and do monthly breast self-exams. There are exceptions to these procedures. Women with increased family risk, those who have had breast cancer, or who have a genetic predisposition to breast cancer should do all the above plus additional tests as the ultrasound and MRI.

Mammography(mammogram): This is an early screening detection tool that uses x-ray compression through image contrasts to identify breast masses and microcalcifications. It actually measures the amount of glandular breast tissue relative to the fatty tissue. Included in all of this fatty tissue is fibrous breast tissue, fat, lobes, lobules, ducts, blood, various types of tissue and calcifications. (It doesn't show cancer in women with large, dense breasts).

Diagnostic Procedures:
AMAS Test-This test detects early breast cancer by identifying malignant growth cells due to its greater sensitivity. If the test is positive you have a mammogram.
Aspirate-A needle is stuck into the lump to withdraw fluid and tissue to identify breast masses and microcalcifications. It actually measures the amount of grandular breast tissue relative to the fatty tissue which is breast density.
Biopsy-Tissue is removed by way of a needle to find out if cells are benign or cancerous from a very suspicious area. This tissue is sent to a lab to be diagnosed by a pathologist. There are different types of biopsies.
Biopsy (Core Steterotactic)-This is a procedure in which they pin point from a

mammogram or ultrasound an area of concern by using a needle to remove the fluid, cells, or tissue to be examined by the pathologist.

CAD (Computer Aided Digital Mammography)-A process where the mammogram is run through a computer to see if there is any missed cancerous tissue.

Scoring of the Mammogram: The mammogram is screened using the CAD (computer aided detection machine) even before the radiologist reads it. This is to see if there are any "false positives," so unnecessary procedures won't be performed.

-The results can be "false negative" where the cancer is missed or even "false positive" where things show up that are not cancerous.

-There are **5 BIRAD scores** for this test and they are: 1, 2, 3, 4, 5.

A one "N" means that the test is negative whereas a score of five "M" means that the test is highly suggestive of a malignancy. Bi-RADS scoring system from the American College of Radiology condensed:

Category O-needs additional evaluation. This is a score from a screening mammogram or one that needs additional testing.

Category 1-negative. The breasts are symmetrical and there are no abnormalities.

Category 2-no cancerous, benign findings. There is no cancer but the radiologist may find a cyst, fibroadenoma or other benign tumor in the breast.

Category 3-probably benign findings, short interval follow-up. This score means you probably have a benign tumor, but to be on the safe side the radiologist recommends a follow-up mammogram after six months.

Category 4-suspicious abnormality, biopsy should be done. This is when a lesion isn't quite cancer, but a biopsy needs to be done to make sure.

Category 5-highly suggestive of malignant cancer and action needs to be taken. This is a lesion that has a high probability of being cancerous and should have a biopsy.

Other Types of Diagnostic Tests Elsewhere in the U.S.- Computerized laser tomography mammography, Electrical Potential Test (using microwave imaging), PET (Positive Emission Tomography), optical imagery, Scientimammography, and Tomosynthesis (digital).

Clinical Breast Exam (CBE)-This is the procedure where the doctor or trained professional exams your breasts and lymph nodes for palpable lumps.

Self Breast Exam or Breast Self Exam (BSE)-A procedure that you should do monthly on your breasts to see if there are any lumps. You should also check your lymph glands.

Thermography- A simple non-invasive test that records the hot heat emissions by way of an infrared light circulating in the breast tissue. It shows inflammation from the heat. Due to this increased circulation, it can detect tumors that can be cancerous five years down the road. Presently there are about a thousand of these machines in the U.S. They are 86-96% accurate.

Types of Mammograms:

Baseline Mammogram-This is a mammogram that is used to identify changes in a women's breast and is used as a measuring guide.

Diagnostic Mammogram-A mammogram usually follows an irregular screening mammogram, if they find a lump, there's a nipple discharge or other skin abnormality.

Screening Mammogram-This mammogram is for women age 40 or above, or who are high risk or there's other genetic concerns.

Ultrasound Sonography(Sonogram)-A painless procedure in which the sonographer uses high frequency sound waves to find abnormalities from mammogram findings. This method can identify solid tumors and fluid filled cysts.

X-Rays Mammograms-Refrain from high dose radiation if you are at risk. Only do low dose mammograms due to the amount of ionizing radiation.

Medical Findings From Tests:

Abscess-Pus collection from a bacterial infection that can occur in the breast.

Adipose Tissue-Fat in the breast tissue.

Atypical Hyperplasia-Tissue that is not like other tissue in that area.

Atypical Lobular Hyperplasia (ALH) and Atypical Ductual Hyperplasia (ADH)- These are extra cells that grow in the ducts, lobules or lobes. They are picked up on mammograms. If you get these you are at strong risk for getting an "active breast" or breast cancer.

Axilla-Under arm, around collar bone and in the chest.

Benign Breast Pain-Treatment can include vitamin E, primrose oil, steroid injections, halting caffeine, diuretics, various hormone pills, and rarely surgery.

Benign Tumors or Masses-A lump or thickened mass area that is not cancerous and often has not spread elsewhere. There can be breast pain with benign tumors. Benign means a negative biopsy and it is not cancerous or malignant.

Breast Density-This is the fat and a measurement of breast density. It's how visible the breast tissue is on mammograms. A patient with dense breasts should have ultrasounds, MRI's and other tests available in their area.

Breast Pain-Ways to reduce breast pain: eat a low fat diet (fruits, vegetables, grains), have cysts drained, learn to relax, limit salt intake, maintain ideal body weight to stabilize hormones, take primrose oil, vitamin E, other vitamins, over the counter pain medicines, watching the caffeine in your diet (pop, coffee, tea) and wearing a supportive bra. Always ask your doctor before taking any pills.

Breast Changes-Breast changes occur over different times in our lives. For example: puberty, menstruation, pregnancy, menopause, and weight changes.

Calcifications, Calcium Deposits or Microcalcifications-These are very small deposits of calcium that you can see on mammograms or ultrasounds. They can be benign 70-80% of the time. Women at age 50 and older are at risk for microcalcifications, clusters of precancerous or cancerous conditions.

Cancer Cells on Mammograms-Cancer cells show up as fuzzy, pointy objects with no clear borders.

Cells-Cells are individual units that make up tissues and organs.

Cyst-A lump that is filled with liquid or a semi solid material.

Dense Breasts-The more x-rays one has the more they will be absorbed and show up as black mammograms. Aggressive cancer can be missed. Mammograms typically pick up calcium deposits and slow moving tumors. That's why ultrasounds and MRI's are important for these women.

Ducts- The hollow channels or hallways in the glands that transport milk from the lobules to the nipple. Cancer in the ducts is more common. This cancer is called infiltrating ductal carcinoma or invasive ductual carcinoma. There is also DCIS which is called ductual carcinoma in situ and is very curable when caught early.

Fibroadenomas - These are cysts that show up as solid, painless, or cancerous cysts or tumors that occur in women between the ages of 18-25. They are granular fibrous tissue that has become firm, hard, can be smooth, or rubbery. These account for 25% of all tumors in women under the ages of 25. They show up as circular oval patches on a mammogram.

Fibrocystic Diet-Eating more fruits, vegetables, grains, legumes, not drinking coffee, eating just a little fat, and taking vitamin E can help with this problem.

Fibrocystic Disease- A benign breast condition that accounts for 80% of all breast cancer due to the abnormalities of hormone levels. The breast can feel lumpy, painful, tender, be swollen, have fluid filled cysts, as well as have a discharge from the nipple.

Hyperplasia-The cells in this area are increased abnormally in number and may occur in the ducts or lobules. If the cells become abnormal, you may get cancer.

Lobes-Each breast has fifteen to twenty lobe sections that contain lobules.

Lobules-These are milk producing glands in the breast that look like a grape stem. Some women get cancer in the lobules. This kind of cancer is called invasive lobular carcinoma or infiltrating lobular carcinoma. It is not a common cancer and often has a poorer prognosis. Another type of cancer in the lobules is called lobular neoplasia or in situ (LCIS) and it is rarely invasive.

Lumps-Seventy-five percent of all lumps women will find while doing a self-exam. A woman should do this exam seven days after the first day of your menstrual cycle.

Lymph-Milky thin fluid that is carried by the lymphatic vessels.

Mastodynia-This is breast pain.

Palpable-This is when you and your doctor can feel the lump.

Pleomorphic-Calcifications that are tiny dots of different sizes and shapes that are linearly arranged. These form in the ducts and can indicate cancer.

Precancer (Premalignant)-A lesion can develop into a malignant neoplasm.

Spiculated-A density that has a starburst shape and is often cancerous.

Types of Benign Cysts/Benign Breast Conditions:

Abscesses-These are pus filled pockets in the breast.

Fat Necrosis-This is when fatty tissue is destroyed in the breast and a lump forms.

Fibrocystic Disease-See above.

Fibroadenoma-See above.

Mammary Dysphasia-This is a barbarous tissue that can increase in size.

Mastitis-Inflammation can cause an infection in the breast. Typically this occurs after breast feeding. Lymph nodes can become swollen, red, warm, lumpy, or tender. Often you have a low grade fever.

Microcalcifications (Calcium Deposits)- We can get tiny calcium deposits or hardened tissue from trauma to the breast, inflammation to the breast, cellular secretions and debris. Most microcalcifications are not cancerous. It's only when they have a certain clumping or clustering pattern on the mammography that additional tests need to be done.

Nodule (Nodulus)-Tissue that is solid and found in a small mass.

Papillomas-These are wart-like growths in the mammary duct by the nipple. They may have a clear or bloody discharge.

Simple Cysts-Simple cysts have no increase in fibrocystic tissue. They are often found in women ages 35-50.

Trauma-Blood can build up in a breast and form a hematoma. A blow or bruise can cause a lump.

Medical Reports:

Mammography report-This is a report of the mammogram procedure.

Radiology report-A sonogram report on the ultrasound.

Surgical pathology report-This is a report that tells the result of a biopsy.

Ultrasound report-A report on the ultrasound procedure.

In the shower:

1 Examine your breasts during bath or shower, when hands glide easier over wet skin. With fingers flat, move firmly over every part of each breast. Use right hand to examine left breast, left hand for right breast. Check for any lump, hard knot, or thickening.

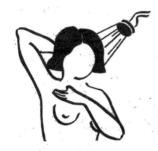

Before a Mirror:

2 Visually inspect your breasts with arms at your sides. Next raise your arms high overhead.

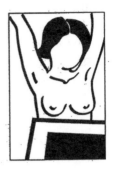

Look for any changes in contour of each breast, a swelling, discharge, dimpling of skin or changes in the nipple.

Then, place hands on hips and press down firmly to flex your chest muscles. Left and right breast will not exactly match—few women's breasts do. Regular inspection shows what is normal for you and will give you confidence in your examination.

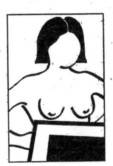

Lying down:

To examine your right breast, put a pillow or folded towel under your right shoulder. Put your right hand behind your head — this

3 spreads the breast tissue evenly over your chest. Use the middle three fingers of your left hand, and keep fingers flat. Press firmly in small circular motion, sliding fingers from one position to the next. Do not lift fingers off the breast until the whole breast is examined. You are feeling for a lump, thickening, or any change which is not normal for you.

Examine the entire breast area including your collarbone, your breast bone, and under your arms.

The diagrams (below) show the three patterns preferred by women and their doctors: the circular (clock) pattern, the vertical strip, and the wedge. Choose the method easiest for you, and use this method each time you examine your breasts.

Finally, *gently* squeeze the nipple of each breast between thumb and index finger. A small amount of waxy discharge in not unusual. Watery or bloody discharge should be reported to your doctor.

After you have completely examined your right breast, examine your left breast using the same method. Compare what you have felt in one breast with the other.

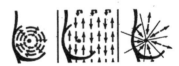

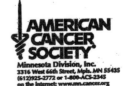

AMERICAN CANCER SOCIETY
Minnesota Division, Inc.
3316 West 66th Street, Mpls. MN 55435
(612)925-2772 or 1-800-ACS-2345
on the internet: www.mn.cancer.org

How To Examine Your Breasts

Lumps Are Not Always Felt By The Finger Tips

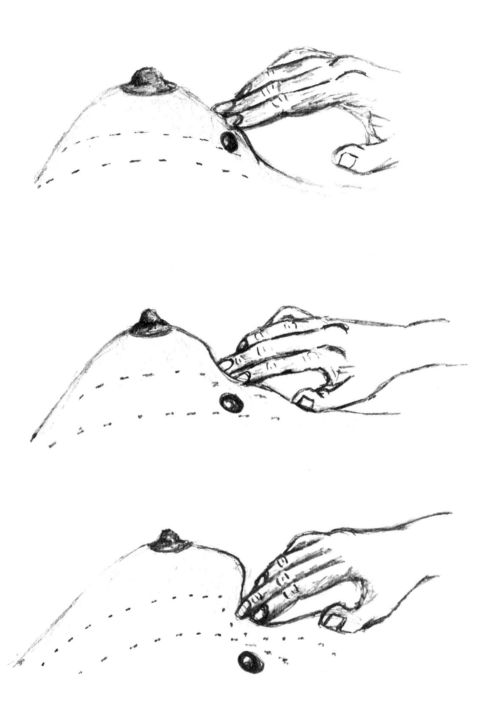

Feel Lymph Gland Areas

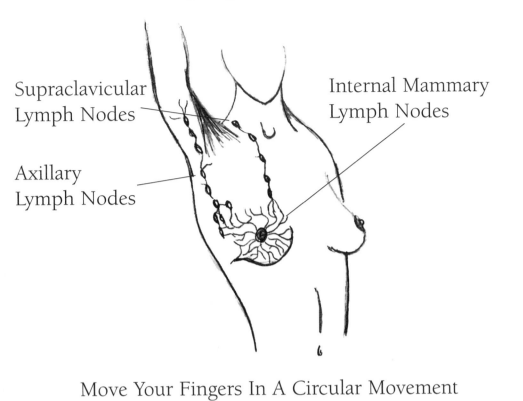

Supraclavicular
Lymph Nodes

Internal Mammary
Lymph Nodes

Axillary
Lymph Nodes

Move Your Fingers In A Circular Movement
Around The Breast Tissue

How Mammography Works

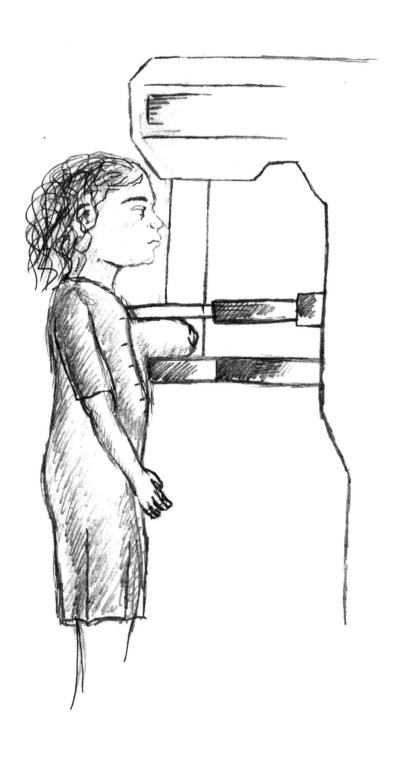

Cross Section of Breast and Lymph Glands

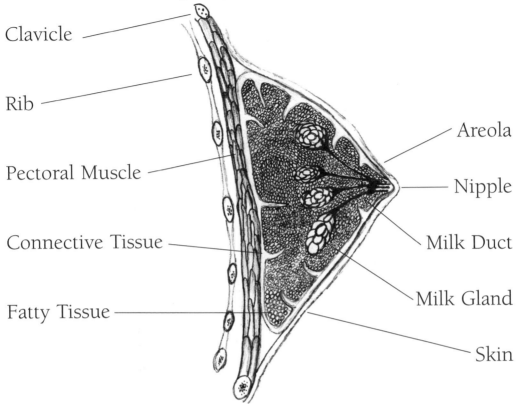

Clavicle

Rib

Pectoral Muscle

Connective Tissue

Fatty Tissue

Areola

Nipple

Milk Duct

Milk Gland

Skin

Lymph Nodes Near The Breast

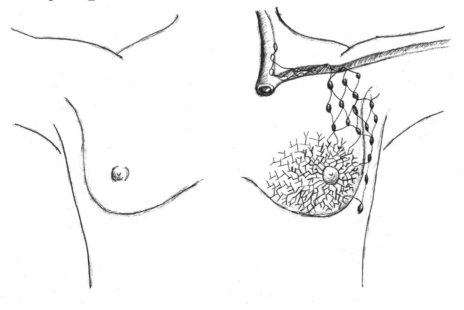

My Breast Screening Guide Chart
I feel this screening guide would save more lives.

Age	Recommendations
Ages 20's and 30's	*Monthly self exams *Clinical breast exam every three years as part of your physical, if you have genetic factors or are in the high risk category *Low dose mammograms if you are in the genetic or high risk category; preferably AMAS testing, thermography ultrasound or breast MRI.
Ages 40-49	*Monthly self exams *Clinical breast exam with a physical each year *Low dose mammogram yearly *Genetic and high risk patients could have AMAS test, thermography, ultrasound, or breast MRI.
Ages 50-74	*Monthly self exams *Clinical breast exam with physicals each year *Low dose mammograms yearly *Genetic and high risk patients could have AMAS test, thermography, ultrasound, or breast MRI.
Ages 75 and older **High Risk**	*Monthly self breast exams *Clinical breast exam yearly or bi-yearly *Low dose mammogram yearly *Talk to your doctor about other screening tools if you are in the high risk category *Those patients with strong family histories or who are a genetic risk could have AMAS test, thermography, ultrasound or breast MRI.

May 12, 2004

Dear Peggy,

Your last letter mentioned a family history of breast cancer. This has stirred up many memories for me.

First, a little background on your great-grandmother Karen Dunne Meier. She was born in Oslo, Norway on Oct. 2, 1862. Grandma Meier immigrated to Minnesota in her teens. My memory is that she came over to help with the children of a family that had previously immigrated from Norway and were living in Grand Marais, MN. In 1881 this family and Grandma, at age 19, moved to Duluth. Eventually she met and married John Meier who at the age of 24, had immigrated from Bergen, Norway in 1886. Incidentally, the story told is that Grandpa Meier came over as John Olson but the immigration official told him that there were too many Olsons here, so he became John Meier.

Grandma and Grandpa built a large house in the West End, across from Lincoln Elementary School on 4th Street, where a community of Norwegians settled. Less than one-half a block away was Zion Lutheran Church built in 1890. Until 1925 all their church services were in Norwegian. But in 1903 the Sunday school started to offer one English class. The Norwegian classes continued until 1932. John started his own moving dray business. Back then that consisted of carts and horses. They had three daughters (Clara, Edna, Jeanette) and five sons (Justin, twins, Bernard and John, Morris and Walford). In 1906 John died of pneumonia at age 43. Grandma was pregnant with her ninth child who was born and died shortly after John's death. Justin, their oldest son, at age 14 started to work on the Lake Superior shipping boats to help support the family.

My Uncle Ben once told me, "All these fancy East End ladies would come in their carriages to have 'Ma' make their dresses." There weren't any racks of dresses back then in the stores, just bolts of cloth. Either you sewed your own or hired a dressmaker. I think she also took in wash and did ironing. Perhaps for those same customers. As the children got old enough some would quit school to help support the family.

Until Grandma went to the hospital for pneumonia and died on April 30, 1942 at the age of 79, I didn't know that she had breast cancer. By then I was almost 14 years old, but people didn't talk about cancer. If it was said, it was a whisper, a subject not discussed until the person died.

It's interesting the things we can recall. I remember how her backyard was almost all garden. The sides and front rows would be full of flowers and the balance vegetables. I suppose that went back to the days when she was raising and feeding a large family.

Grandma had been a widow for thirty-six years and raised eight children by herself in a country far from her birth. I think this is amazing.

Next week, I'll write about your Grandma Edna Prahl, my Mom's story of breast cancer.

Love always,

Aunt Karen

May 17, 2004

Dear Peggy,

This morning I went to my Lung Power Rehabilitation group. I spent 20 minutes on the treadmill and 20 minutes on the "NuStep," a bike that you pedal and pull the handle bars back and forth. When I was first recommended to this group by my doctor in 1999, my blood oxygen level range was 91-92. If it drops below 90, I need to be on full time oxygen. It took me about six months of exercising and learning to live with COPD to get that level to move up. Now, unless I have an infection, it's usually 94-96.

Today is a good day for me to finish our family history regarding breast cancer. Your Grandmother's (Edna Meier Prahl) first round of cancer was in 1936. She was 37 years old and I was 8. One morning as I was leaving for school, she told me, "Grandma Meier will be at our house after school as I have to go to the hospital for an operation." Years later I learned that the surgeon, our family physician and friend, did a mastectomy and took her back to surgery a few days later to try to get all the cancer. The doctor told Dad he was sorry but he couldn't get all of it all. Dad was also told to hire a housekeeper to raise his children. However, as Mom regained her strength at home she started getting up earlier and earlier to get the house straightened up, and the beds made before the housekeeper arrived. She didn't want anyone to ever see her home messy. Dad finally realized that having a housekeeper was difficult on Mom. The day finally came when Mom was back in charge.

I thought all was well. She had surgery, lost a breast, and I wasn't aware of her poor prognosis. That is until sometime in the summer of 1937 when I must of spoken back to Mom. Dad got angry and took me out on the front steps of our Hunter's Park home to scold me and said, "Mom is dying of cancer and you should behave." In the 4th grade at Washburn, our teacher said she was going to call Marylu's and my Mother when we got into trouble. I blurted out that she couldn't because, "My Mother is dying of cancer." I think that may have been the only time I ever used the word cancer or heard it used in regards to my Mom until 1952. Dad never talked about this incident again. As the years passed I decided that he had made that up to get me to behave. Now in looking back, I realize what a burden he had to carry. He knew what the doctor had told him, and he dearly loved his wife.

Mom was always physically active. In the winter she played volleyball in the evenings each week at Washburn School. These games were later replaced by weekly bowling. She also ice skated every week in the winter at the Duluth Curling Club. In the summer she played golf weekly with two ladies groups. One day she was at the Pike Lake Auto Club Golf course and a different day at Ridgeview Country Club. Many weekends both Dad and her would golf with friends.

In spite of all her sporting activities, she always had time for her church's active Ladies Aid Society and their Guild, holding many offices. She was a life member of ELC Women's Missions, a Red Cross volunteer for many years, WWII air warden for our block and took part in many activities supporting our community.

I now wonder how she could fit it all in along with raising two children, keeping a spic and span house, cooking well balanced meals, sewing, family get-togethers and other entertaining. In the winter she would sew her golf dresses for the next season. In the fall those dresses became her "housedresses." Back then women didn't wear pants or jeans. She sewed many outfits for me and was always ready to help a friend or family member.

Remember when I said that no one talked about cancer until someone died from it? There were few, if any books on the disease that the general public read. It wasn't like today where our library shelves are full of books on cancer. Magazines, newspapers, the internet, and the TV can tell us much about the disease.

To my knowledge after our family physician died, she didn't go to the doctor. Chemo or radiation wasn't an option back then. She was leading a very busy and interesting life.

In 1952 Mom and I were traveling around Florida and she mentioned to me that she thought she should see a doctor as she hadn't for so many years. Since she seemed fine to me, I assumed for a check up. She asked for suggestions on who to see, and I told her who my boyfriend Jim's parents went to. He was a well respected internal medicine doctor in the Medical Arts Building. After we got home, she called and got an appointment for March 7, 1952. Her long remission was over.

But, before I forget it, Aunt Clara, Mom's oldest sister, died from breast cancer. She received this diagnosis at age 58, had a mastectomy and died four years later. Her granddaughter, Terry got cervical cancer in her 20's and died at age 36 of metastatic breast cancer.

On my Dad's side, neither his mother or his three sisters ever had cancer. As far as I know, none of their children did either. Enough family history for today.

Love,

Aunt Karen

Present Breast Screening Recommendations:

American Cancer Society: Clinical Breast Exam-Every 3 years between ages 20-39. Every year beginning at age 40.   Breast Self-Exam-Beginning at age 20 you should discuss a self-breast exam with your family physician. Mammography-If you are ages 40-70 and older you should have a mammogram each year.

National Cancer Institute: Clinical Breast Exam-Every year starting at age 30. Breast Self-Exam-There is no recommendation. Mammography-Every year from ages 40 on.

U.S. Preventative Services: Clinical Breast Exam-There is no recommendation for having this done or not having it done. Breast Self-Exam-There is no recommendation either way on this matter. Mammography-Every one to two years depending on the health of the individual patient.

Susan G. Kromen Breast Cancer Foundation: Clinical Breast Exam-Every three years between the ages of 20-39. Every year after age 39. Breast Self-Exam-This should be every month starting at age 20. Mammography-This should be every year starting at age 40 and beyond.

Free Mammograms For Those Who Qualify:
   Those women who qualify can get free mammograms through the YWCA Breast Awareness Program (1-800-815-8298), and The Sage Screening Program through the Minnesota Department of Health (1-888-643-2584).

"Cherish each day as a priceless gift."   -Abbey Press

"For everything on earth has it's own time and it's own season."   -Ecclesiastes 3:1

"Most growth is accompanied by pain. Better to have suffered and grown than never to have suffered at all. God can use heartache as well as headache to help us grow."
      -Author Unknown

"Life is a succession of lessons which must be lived to be understood."   -Helen Keller

"Hold fast to dreams, for if dreams die, life is a broken-winged bird that cannot fly."
      -Langston Hughes

6/11/04

Dear Auntie Karen,

How's my number one cheerleader doing today? I'm so delighted that you are making an appointment at the University of Minnesota Hospital to see someone about your respiratory fungal infection. God knows you have suffered long enough with this, and your quality of life needs improvement. You've gone from almost dying to your present state. Who would think that corticosteroids that you need to breathe and live with for COPD would be like a double-edged sword. I'm almost afraid to use my asthma inhaler. But I guess after almost 10 years of use some complications are inevitable.

Today we are experiencing fair weather in upstate Minnesota and it's allowed Jim and I to get a few things done around here before going to the Duluth Clinic. Jim will have more time to do things around the house as his last day of work at Central High School was Friday. He loves teaching part-time, being retired and his students keep him young. Jim is already making plans for a summer job, as he likes to keep busy and enjoys the interaction with so many people.

Life is certainly full of salt and pepper. No matter what memories seem to tie you to your family, there are pleasant and not so pleasant ones. My kids forever amaze me. They both have minds of their own and their stressors become mine. I hope I'm not making myself sick by their choices. They need to learn by their own mistakes. At times, I forget that I learned from my own mistakes. Some times it's hard to separate being a teacher and a parent. I internalized a lot of stress being a teacher wearing the stress around my collar and sleeves, but I am no longer a teacher and try to be a parent at arm's length.

It's our heart's desire now that we are retired to make changes to our aged house, so we won't have any future problems. Dave Twining has finished the electrical work on two of our garages. The swimming pool is grounded for the first time in twenty-eight years. We had our gutters fixed and replaced. The Woodland Hills Cougars will be coming tomorrow to dig up my flower garden as I want a permanent garden of bushes and flowers. Miller Roofing is fixing our roof. Our neighbor, Charlene, former East High School secretary, took a picture of the men working on the roof. She called the picture "Fiddler on the Roof." We still have a lot to get ready, so the furniture can be moved out of the house and the oak floors redone. It will all happen in due time, but this worry about cancer complicates our plans.

I hope all is well in out sized Minneapolis. Is Uncle Jim sticking to his diabetic diet? Right? The twins must be due soon. I hope Shannon is coping with being bedridden and the medical problems that go along with this pregnancy. My heart goes out to Shannon. A Central teacher went through some similar medical problems last year. Jeff must be exhausted starting a new program for Anoka County dealing with families with multiple issues and needs, going to school to get his master's, and moving to a new home. Life brings with it many trials and joys along the way.

Today I went for my second ultrasound at the clinic. My first this year was done on May 12, 2004. I don't know if I told you that this exam was "normal." It went on to state that "A negative mammogram does not exclude the possibility of breast disease. You should never ignore a breast lump or any other change in the breasts even if the mammogram is normal." (There's strong evidence that rigorous training and experience helps radiologists to read mammograms better. Now they have the

CAD to pre-read it for them.) My next mammogram is scheduled for May 12, 2005 on the left breast. I haven't had one on the right breast for quite some time. This was a form letter except for a few dates. Sounds like we have to be our own advocate, but I'm the first to say that I have a whole lot to learn.

My ultrasound this time went favorably well. I had a great ultrasound sonographer named Roma. She skillfully did my whole breast very thoroughly. This was not like my earlier ultrasound where only half the breast was done, and I was in and out very quickly. If you recall, a nurse told me to go home, put a piece of tape on the lump, measure it periodically and then go back to my doctor if I had any concerns. I came home on that day and said to Jim "What the heck! I found a lump and went to my doctor. Dr. Nisswandt sent me for an ultrasound, but I ended up with half an ultrasound, but I can still feel the lump." Jim's reply was one of confusion as he could feel it as well, yet he didn't want to make any assumptions. I was depending on health professionals to find the problem. I still didn't have an answer to the lump. The sonographer this time was very thorough. Thank goodness some are so dedicated and accurate!

Also, today I had a biopsy right after the ultrasound was done. Roma, the sonographer, got Dr. Hoyer who after checking the ultra sound results, did a biopsy immediately. I think the radiologist can only be as good as the sonographer that does their job first. Dr. Hoyer, a detailed oriented doctor, did this biopsy on the spot as he has an eye for breast cancer. He put a metal clip in my breast. During this process my blood pressure went up as I thought, "Why me?" I had a bad feeling about this, call it my intuition. After this I had a mammogram of my left breast. I realize that eighty percent of all breast tumors are benign, but I also know that women are at risk of developing breast cancer. I've read that breast cancer is the second leading cause of death in women. Waiting for the results is a woman's worst nightmare. It's the fear of the big "BC".

I found a piece of paper from a workshop that I went to in 1986. It said I weighed

120 pounds. Now I weigh 189 pounds and I'm one "chunky monkey." To think that I use to weigh 85-92 pounds in college and had eating issues. I found another medical report which stated my triglycerides were 413 in 2003. I really believe my diet isn't the best. We eat the way we are raised. Meat was the basis of the meal. I've eaten too many saturated fats such as potato chips and sugar coated licorice which I love. My diet is very high in red meat, dairy and especially cheese. It's low in fruits, grains and vegetables because I've never cared for these kinds of food. I drink one drink a year and don't smoke.

God must have something else in mind for me. Why has he chosen me? All I can think is "Lord just get me through this uncertainty."

Affectionately,

Peggy

P.S. Here is our new medical lesson that includes some pictures of biopsies, fibrocystic breasts, milk producing lobules, and a draft of a risk chart I made.

Symptoms and Risk Factors for Breast Cancer, Diagnostic Tests, Cancerous Medical Findings and Reports

Cancer Facts, Terms, Knowledge, Concepts

Symptoms/Risk Facts For Breast Cancer:

There are many risk factors for breast cancer that come from different sources:

1.Age-Increasing age puts all women at risk for breast cancer.

2.Alcohol Consumption and Smoking-Drug usage can place you at a higher risk. One or more drinks per day is risky.

3.Birth-When you haven't given birth before age 30 or haven't given birth, you are at an increased risk.

4.Breast Implants and Dense Breasts-Implants and dense breasts can place you at a higher risk for breast cancer.

5.Contraceptives-Long term use of contraceptives may put women at risk.

6.DES (Diethylstilbesterol)-This was a drug prescribed to women between the years of 1940-71 to prevent pregnancy complications. It is a strong cause for increased risk for breast cancer in the daughters of the women who took it.

7.Family Cancer History-A family history of breast cancer can put women at risk. Also when a first degree relative as a mother, sister, or grandmother gets breast cancer it increases your chances. This tendency accounts for 5% of all breast cancers. Premenopausal women have to be cautious.

8.Gender-If you are a woman you are at risk, but men can get breast cancer as it can run in families and is increasing.

9.Genetic-BRCA1, BRCA2 are genetic indicators of breast cancer. They are tied to cancers that run in families as ovary, thyroid, colon, and endometrial cancer. If you have this gene, you may have a lifetime risk of 35-85% in developing breast cancer. With these genes you should consider a total bilateral mastectomy and your ovaries removed after genetic counseling. This gene accounts for 5% of all cancers. (Genetic testing is important for families with BRCA 3, Noey 2, thyroid cancer, Aderomatous polyposis, breast cancer, ovarian cancer, Li Frameri Syndrome, p.53, BARDI, Wilm's tumors and Tetinoblastoma.)

10.High Fat; Low Fiber, Fruits and Vegetable Diet-Red meat is injected with hormones as well as poultry that puts women at a higher risk for breast cancer. Women need to eat a high fiber, high fruit, high vegetable diet like our ancestors.

12.Hormone Pills-Long term use of HTR (estrogen or progesterone replacement) therapy may put women at risk. These women may have too much estrogen or progesterone circulating in their blood. There is evidence linking it to breast cancer but it is not the sole cause.

13.Life Style Choices-Factors as drinking one drink or more per day or some environmental toxins can put some women at risk.

14.Menstruation and Menopause-If a girl gets her period at a young age (9-12), this may increase her risk for breast cancer. A long menstrual history, one that starts early or ends late in life as menopause after age 55 are also risk factors.

15.Obesity-If you have a lot of fat you are at risk because of the larger amounts of circulating hormones in your stored fat. Studies show that both pre and postmenopausal overweight women are more likely to die from this disease. Other studies state being overweight after menopause or gaining weight as an adult are factors.

16.Previous History of Breast Cancer-If you have had breast cancer you are at a higher risk for recurrence. Atypical hyperplasia, biopsy confirmed hyperplasia and in situ can put a woman at risk.

17.Race-Caucasian women are at higher risk for breast cancer. African American women have higher fatality rates because they don't seek treatment early enough. Hispanic, Native American and Asian women have a lower incident rate of breast cancer. Native Americans have a higher fatality rate from not seeking treatment. Ashkenazi Jews have a 1 out of 40 chance of developing breast cancer.

18.Radiation-If a woman has had high doses of ionizing radiation before age 35, she may be at risk for breast cancer later in life. Ironizing radiation is the only environmental factor proven to cause breast cancer. If a woman has low-dose ionizing radiation in mid life this can put her at risk.

Hot Flashes-Avoid foods that trigger hot flashes as spicy foods, activities that involve heat, alcohol, and daily stressors. Dress lightly or in layers, carry cold water with you, bring a mini fan in your purse, and learn to relax. Some people take vitamin E, take black cohosh, and eat foods high in phytoestrogens. Doctors can prescribe any of the following pills: Efflexor, Prozac, Neurontin, Megace, Depro-Provera shots, and Catapres. **Always consult your doctor first.**

Diagnostic Procedures:

Core Biopsy (Mammotomy)-The radiologist performs a simple procedure by taking a larger area of tissue from your breast and sends it to the pathology lab to be examined. This procedure is often done using an ultrasound. There are **two types**:

1.Sterotactic Core Needle Biopsy-An area of concern where tissue is removed that has been pinpointed by way of a mammogram.

2.Ultrasound Guided Core Biopsy-A biopsy where they use the ultrasound and the waves are outlined at the site that have a solid mass.

Ductual Lavage-Fluid is taken out of the duct. A few centers use this procedure and it reduces breast cancer by forty five percent.

Ductography (Galactography)-A catheter is put into the duct, dye injected and an x-ray taken.

Early Breast Cancer Diagnosis-Breast cancer can be prevented if women and men do self-exams each month, clinical breast exams and mammograms once a year. Tumors are: benign (negative) and malignant (positive).

Fine Needle Biopsy-This is when a very thin needle is used under local anesthesia to see if a lump or mass is cancerous. The fluid is taken out and if it disappears it is not cancerous. The tissue is then sent to the lab. This procedure has the highest rate of false negative results.

Kinder Biopsies- These include Mammotone breast biopsy, ultrasound probe, x-rays and procedures that vacuum the tissues.

Preventing Breast Cancer-Breast cancer can be prevented by exercise, maintaining a healthy life style by managing stressors, keeping a healthy weight, and taking nutritional supplements if your diet is lacking in nutrients.

Medical Findings:

Biopsy risk: Hematoma-A collection of blood can form at the biopsy site that often is absorbed into the blood. There may be a visible scar or scar tissue that makes future mammograms hard to read accurately.

BRCA1-This is a hereditary gene located on the 17th chromosome. It's a gene that makes you at risk for inheriting breast and ovarian cancer. Commonly found in Ashkenazi Jewish descendants.

BRCA2-Another hereditary gene located on 13th chromosome. It increases your risk for breast cancer. Commonly found in Ashkenazi Jewish descendants.

Breast Reduction-Breast reduction can help large breasted women from getting cancer if they have dense breasts.

Cancer-The uncontrolled growth of cells in the body that grow, invade, and destroy surrounding tissue.

Carcinogenic-This means cancer causing.

Carcinoma-Cancerous tumors that show a growth of abnormal cells in the breast tissue resulting from a malignancy or lump that has grown.

DCIS Cases -These are 50% of the cases where microcalcifications (clusters of tiny grains of calcium) can be seen on a mammogram. They go undetected until they become malignant or you have a biopsy. The question is whether to treat the DCIS cases as radically as invasive is a topic of debate. Some DCIS doesn't turn into cancer.

Ductual Carcinoma-The most common type of breast cancer.

Ductual Carcinoma in Situ (DCIS)-Cancer that is contained in the ducts and shows up as poorly shaped white sand on a mammogram. Some will become invasive. There are different grades: I, II, and III.

Familial Cancer-Cancer that occurs more frequently than by chance in a family.

Genetic-This has to do with your genes and hereditary characteristics.

Incident of Breast Cancer-Research according to the A.C. S. shows that 80% of all breast cancer occurs in the ducts and 20% occurs in the breast lobes. Breast cancer can be fatal if not treated. It can occur in the breast, in the lymph nodes, or metastasize elsewhere in the body.

Inflammatory Breast Cancer-This is a less common cancer that occurs 1-1.5% of the time. It clogs the channels and symptoms include increased breast size with density, redness, warmth, swelling, constant pain, and an orange like skin called peau'd orange. An individual that has this kind of cancer needs aggressive surgery and chemo.

Invasive Breast Cancer (also Infiltrating BC)-This is cancer that has spread outside its site of origin to infiltrate through the ducts or lobules into the connective or fatty tissue.

Invasion-The cancerous mass moves between the normal cells.

Invasive Infiltrating Lobular Carcinoma (IL)-A cancer that grows in the lobule walls and spreads. It's not a common type of cancer and occurs in 10% of the cases.

Lobular Carcinoma in Situ (LCIS)-This is irregular cells that grow in the lining wall of the lobule. It can't be felt and often is picked up on a biopsy. This happens 1% of the time with women.

Lymph Node Cancer Symptoms-Signs of cancer are non-movable glands that can show up as bumpy, tender, hard, enlarged, and may not change in size. They may be connected to other nodes.

Malignant Tumors-A cancerous tumor that lines the duct or lobes of the breast. If it doesn't leave the ducts or lobes its non-invasive. It can be in situ as well. The tumor can have uncontrolled growth (metastasizes) or invasion outside of the duct or lobe.

Medullary Carcinoma-A less common cancer that shows up in 1-7% of the breast cancer cases. It has a better prognosis than ductual or lobular carcinoma.

Metastasize-This is when new cancer cells spread to a different site. If cancer is caught in the early stages it won't metastasize.

Mucinous-A less common cancer.

Multifocal-Breast Cancer that is on one or more lobes or ducts.

Non-Cancerous Lymph Node-This is a lymph node that doesn't change in size, is movable, has a smooth, soft touch, and is very tender when enlarged. It often is more isolated with clear areas.

Paget's Disease-Erosion of the breast nipple with cancer cells. Often the symptoms are crustiness and oozing.

Papillary Carcinoma-A less common breast cancer that has finger like projections and is often common in situ cancer. Sometimes it becomes invasive. Occurs in 2.5% of all invasive cancers.

Primary Tumor-Site where the cancer has started.

Polygenic Breast Cancer- These are cases where breast cancer doesn't run in a family but most members develop the disease. There's a 3.3 lifetime risk of getting it if you are a family member.

Post menopausal-This is the time after menopause when you have no menstrual periods. The time period is your late 40's and early 50's.

Pre menopausal-A time before menopause when you have menstrual cycles.

Secondary Tumor-The second place in which a tumor is found.

Sporadic Breast Cancer-This is when there is no known history of breast cancer.

Tubular Carcinoma-A less common cancer that occurs in 1-2% of all breast cancers, has a better prognosis, and rarely metastasizes.

Biopsies

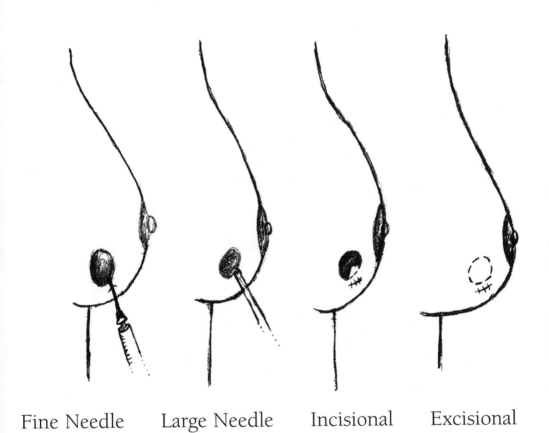

Fine Needle   Large Needle   Incisional   Excisional

Needle Biopsies   Open Biopsies

Fibrocystic Breasts

Fibrocystic Breasts are often associated with women's hormonal changes.

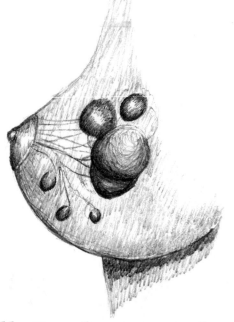

Milk Producing Lobules

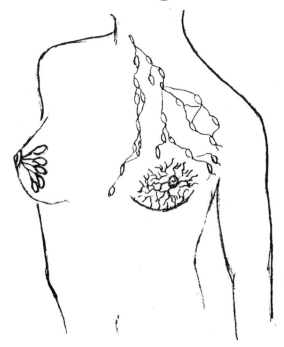

Hereditary and Non-Hereditary Risk Factors Chart

Factor Type	Risk

Individual and Genetic Factors:

Family History of Breast Cancer   Large Risk

Women who come from families with first degree relatives who have had breast cancer, account for 5-10% of all breast cancers. Other sources state that familial breast cancer involving a mother or a sister can increase your risk for breast cancer up to 50%. These women need to be monitored by several diagnostic procedures.

BRCA1 and BRCA2 /Others   Large Risk

There is convincing evidence that there is an association with a large increase in breast cancer when you carry genetic genes. BRCA1 and BRCA2 account for 5% of all breast cancers. If you have BRCA1 you have a 35-85% chance of getting breast cancer. If a family member gets ovarian cancer it is often a signal of genetic cancer. Research has identified other defective genes that contribute to breast cancer. They include BRCA3 and Noey 2 from the father's side, CDKN2A; (p.53) Li Fraumers Sydrome (a rare breast cancer), Ataxia telangiectasia (a mutant gene that accounts for 1% of all breast cancers), and PTEN gene (Cowden's syndrome).

Increasing Age   (Over 50)   Very Large Risk

There's convincing evidence that increasing age puts women at risk. More than 75% of breast cancers occur in women older than 50. Women over 40 have an 18% chance of getting breast cancer, and women under 30 have a 1.5% chance of getting breast cancer.

Gender   Very Large Risk

There's convincing evidence that there is a very large association with an increase in breast cancer risk among females. Men have a 1% risk and often if is from genetics or a strong family history of cancer.

Race   Specific Ethnicity: High Risk

Caucasian women are at the highest incident rate. (SEERS)- "The life time risk of getting invasive breast cancer for all races is 13.39%, 14.21% for Caucasians, and 9.99% for blacks." The American Cancer society states in their literature that, "1 out 7 women will get invasive breast cancer in their life time." The National Cancer Institute states, "**African American** women have a higher incident **death rate** for not seeking treatment early enough." Other sources state, 1 out of every 40 Ashkenazi Jewish women, of Eastern European decent, will get breast cancer. Asians, Hispanics, and Native Americans have a lower incident rate of getting breast cancer according to several sources.

Height   Moderate Risk

Women taller than five feet, nine inches have a moderate increased risk for breast cancer. A study of 10,000 women found that women who reached their full height at age 13 or younger, reflected higher estrogen levels due to bone building mass, bone density, and growth. This maybe due to genetics, nutrition or hormonal levels.

Reproductive/Female Factors:

Birth   **Moderate Risk**

There is convincing evidence that there is a moderate association risk with birth. If a women does not have a child and doesn't breast feed before age 30, she is at risk.

Atypical Hyperplasia, Fibrocystic or Benign Proliferate Breast Disease, or Hyperplasia In Situ   **Large Risk**

There is convincing evidence that there is an association with a large increase in breast cancer when atypical hyperplasia follows a biopsy. The spreading of cells can put a woman at a one and half time risk in comparison to other women. A previous biopsy can put a woman at increased risk by four to five times in comparison to other woman.

Early Menstruation Cycle, Late Menopause   **Moderate Risk**

There is convincing evidence that there is moderate increases in breast cancer risk. If a girl starts menstruating at age 12 or younger, she may be at risk for later breast cancer in comparison to a girl who menstruates at ages 14-16 years of age. If a woman has late menopause at age 55 or later, she may be at risk for breast cancer compared to a women at age 45.

DES (Diethylstilbestrol)   **Slightly Associated Risk**

Women took this medication in the past to prevent miscarriages, and their daughters may be at risk for breast cancer according to some sources.

Breast Implants   **Associated Risk**

Women who have breast implants wrapped in polurethane foam maybe at risk for breast cancer according to some sources.

Dense Breasted Women   **Large Risk**

Women who have dense breasts are at risk for breast cancer. Density might not be related to breast size. There has been studies of small women with large breasts and tall women with dense breasts. Density is how dark the mammogram is and seeing the susceptible cells. Mammograms don't pick up fast growing tumors. These women may need tomography, AMAS testing, ultrasounds, and (or) MRI's.

Oral Contraceptives   **Moderate Risk**

There is convincing evidence of moderate increases in breast cancer risk by taking oral contraceptives. Especially if a women took OC's before 1975. Other factors are how early the individual started using contraceptives and at what age.

Hormone Pills/HRT (Estrogen Replacement Therapy)   **Moderate Risk**

There is convincing evidence of a moderate increase in breast cancer risk from using HRT. Estrogen with progestin puts a women at an individual risk for breast cancer due to increased breast density. There is a life time risk from using HRT after menopause. There are many advantages of HRT for many women. The level of estrogen dominance in the body can determine breast cancer incident. Premarin R and Prempo increases a woman's chances of getting breast cancer. There are better choices as Orthrit for replacement therapy. There's an estrogen metabolism C-16 molecule that puts some women at high risk. These women should use diet and exercise to reduce their risk.

Previous History of Breast Cancer, Lobular Carcinoma In Situ   High Risk

If you have had cancer in one breast, it will increase your chances of getting it in another breast by three to four times. Lobular in situ increases your chances of breast cancer.

Life Style Factor Choices:

High Socioeconomic Position   Moderate Risk

Obesity, Being Overweight   Moderate Risk

Women who are obese after menopause have a higher incident rate of breast cancer and it increases their chances ten fold. The ovaries are no longer producing as much estrogen as the adrenal glands. The hormones are stored in the fat and circulating hormones and the fat cells metasize into estrogen. Women who are overweight have a higher and longer exposure added to HRT. These women have a higher chance of dying from breast cancer.

Diet--High Fatty Meats and Dairy; Low Fiber, Fruits, Vegetables, Grains

**   High Risk by Some Sources**

There are studies being done on high red meat ingestion, cured meats, well done meats, high dairy, consumption of soy products, fiber, and phytoestrogens. The data is up and down on hormones. Red meat holds more controversy. There may not be enough studies done on dairy, chicken, and fish. Harvard Medical School claims 30% of all cancer deaths are from food. Other sources feel diet plays a role in breast cancer, hormones, and obesity.

Fatty meats have 17 beta estradiols and other strong steroids in them. Synthetic estrogens as Zeranol are implanted in beef cattle and are known as endocrine disruptors. Heifers are fed Melengesterol acetate, a synthetic progesterone for birth control that promotes weight gain. These xenohormones act like estrogen in the body. Bovine growth hormones used for dairy milk production are endocrine disruptors as well and have been linked to breast cancer. Remember animal fat retains pesticides and environmental toxins.

Organochlorines (DDT and chlorine) are found in fish, birds, and livestock in their fatty tissues as well as in corn, grains and milk. Foods we eat contain pesticides, mercury, PCB's, DDE, TDE, Phthalates, biphenyl A, and dioxins. Several sources feel they are in one's circulating hormones, in our stored body fat, in dairy products, breast milk, and animal fats that we consume.

Fish need to come from oceans, be wild, be smaller (with less storage). Always check the mercury levels of various fish.

Lack of Exercise and a Sedentary life Ltyle   Large Risk

The American Cancer Society states in their literature that, "vigorous activity 5 days or more per week, may further enhance reduction in breast and colon cancer."

Smoking   Potential but Controversial Risk

There are studies underway about heavy smoking and heavy exposure to smoking. Harvard Medical Studies claim that 30% of the cancer deaths are from smoking.

34

Stress   **Contributing Factor**

Stress does not cause cancer but it effects hormones that have an effect on the cancerous condition.

Alcohol   **Moderate Risk**

There is convincing evidence of an association with moderate increases in breast cancer risk. Women who drink more than one drink a day are more at risk for breast cancer. You increase your risk by 21% according to ACS. They also state "regular consumption of even a few drinks per week has been associated with increased risk for breast cancer in women." Women who drink excessively lack folic acid in their diets often times.

Dark Hair Dye   **Risk Being Studied**

A woman is at risk because of coal tar dyes, lead acetate, phenylene, and other xenohormones. They are probably human carcinogens.

Cosmetics, Shampoos, Conditioners, Make-up, Nail Polish   **Potential Risk**
Some Deodorants, Antiperspirants   **No Association Risk**

Deodorants and antiperspirants have been found in breast tumors and studies have shown no breast cancer association. Benzyl violet 4B, formaldehyde, dibutyl phthalate(DBP), selenium sulfide are just a few listed as known and probable human carcinogens found in nail treatments, hair removal creams, facial cleaners, nail polish, sun screens, sun oils, and shampoos. Other sources state parabens and xenohormones products, and they have been found in women's breast tumors.

Previous Mammograms Treatments and Other Procedures   **Very Large Risk**

There is convincing evidence that there is a very large increase in breast cancer risk from having repeated mammograms early on in younger women. Mammograms can increase deaths in these cases only. Women who have mammograms when older are not at risk. Mammograms now days are low ionizing radiation whereas years ago they were high dose which weakened the immune system. There are critical periods in radiation susceptibility. For example, if your breast has been exposed to radiation before age five, you increase your chances. Harvard Medical Report states women are only at a 1% risk for having mammograms and other diagnostic procedures today.

Ironizing Radiation   **Risk Depends on Exposure Age**

Most places no longer have high dose ionizing radiation on x-rays. A woman could have been exposed to high dose in the past, and it could increase her risk today. It's good to ask. Thermography and MRI are low dose. If a child is exposed to radiation for scoliosis at a young age, this can increase risk by nine fold. The National Cancer has done a study on ionizing radiation.

Environmental Factors:

Pesticides   **Possible Risk**

DDT and DDE increase estrogenic activity by suppressing the immune system. Chlorinated organic and organchlorines in pesticides are a BC risk. They effect body fat and breast tissues as well as being found in animal and fish fat. Bananas and strawberries have pesticides on them, to name just a few fruits. Always cook, peel, wash, trim foods, and eat a wide variety of organic foods. Like all chemicals it would depend on continual exposure.

Charcoal

Chemicals   Possible Risk

Certain chemicals can possibly cause breast cancer. They include: estrogens, progestins, solvents, polycyclic aromatic hydrocarbons (PAH's), 1,3-butadiene and aromatic amines. In other words these include hormone pills, p-nonylphenol that is used in plastics as well as other xenoestrogens such as BPA. Tufts University has done research in this area as well as other research sites. You find BPA's in baby bottles, the lining of metal cans as well as plastic containers that leach chemicals. PVC's are also found in food packaging, medical products, credit cards, and even rainwear. PVC's have been linked to increased death for breast cancer among workers who are employed in the production of these products. Pesticides as aldrin and dieldrin have been used on crops and are in the soil. Organchlorine compounds were diagnosed in many breast tumors. There are many household products that mimic estrogen and cause mammary cancer in lab animals. Industrial solvents have been implicated in lab tumors. There is also 1,3-butadiene that is found in feedstock, tobacoo smoke, and is created by internal combustion engines and petroleum refineries. These have caused mammary tumors in lab animals. Lastly there is aromic amines that are found in plastic and include tobacco smoke, grilled meats and fish. They are also found in rivers, air, cigarette smoke, disiel exhaust, and in various combustion sites.

Herbicides   Possible Risk

There are few studies done on 2, 4-D which are suspected endocrine disruptors. These are also found in drinking water, is the most widely used herbicide used in the U.S. and was even used in Agent Orange. Workers who manufacture these products or are involved with treatment products are at risk. They may include pesticide applicators, agricultural, forestry workers, laundry workers. Farmers who work with 2, 4-D have weakened their immune systems. There are few studies on chemical exposure though.

Radon   Unlikely Risk

Radon would have to hit the blood stream and other parts of the body before entering the breast, so it is unlikely that it is a cause of breast cancer. It's wise to test your home for radon though.

Air, involuntary inhalation   Uncertain Risk

Avoid high ozone levels by not exercising outside or being out on these days.

Water   Uncertain Risk

Atrazine, Cyanzine, simazine, alachlor and metolachlor which are applied to crops drain into lakes, rivers and the ground supply. Water can have acute water borne diseases, toxic bacteria, lead (that accumulates in the body) and pesticides that are linked to cancer. Atrazine and Simazine are often found in water. Nitrates and nitrites from human and animal waste, and field fertilizers are found in water. High levels of chlorine as well as chloroform are found in water. There may also be formeldyhate in the water. Home water testing and filtration are important.

36

Sunlight   Unlikely Risk

Excessive sunlight and not being protected can cause damage to DNA that can
let cancer get into the body system. Bad genes modify bad genes and set the
environmental triggers off.

Nuclear Sources   Possible Risk, Uncertain
Where you work   Risky Professions

Women or men who work in petrochemical plants or electrical workers are at
higher risk. If you work with vinyl chloride you have an increased risk for breast
cancer. A variety of professions are being studied as well as working the night shift
and levels of melatonin. There are several areas of employment that are under study.
They include: lab, biomedical, cosmetologists, semi-conductor workers, printers,
textile dying, airline personnel, health care workers, and metal plate workers.
Work place risks include the using of acid mists, benzene, carbon tetrachloride,
ethylene oxide, formaldehyde, lead oxide, ethylene chloride, and styrene.

Where you live   Uncertain Risk

Where you live can increase your risk for breast cancer. If a person lives near a
nuclear power plants, power plants, or hazardous toxic waste facilities, there have been
excessive deaths due to breast cancer in these areas.

Other electromagnetic fields   Unlikely, But Under Study

Magnetic fields are under study. If a home has high electrical fields, EMF exposure,
it can reduce pineal glands production of melatonin resulting in mammary cancer. An
environmental testing company can test for EMF exposure. Other magnetic fields can
include microwaves, TV's, and hair dryers.

Place of Residence   Large Risk

Women who live in Northern America,Western and Northern Europe are at increased
risk.

Sources of Information: Breast Cancer and Environmental Risk Factors-Sprecher Institute of Comparative,
Breast Cancer Fund and Breast Cancer Action Book, and a variety of **other numerous sources**.

Risks are based on large numbers of women with the disease or exposure in comparison to large numbers
without the disease. It's group risk, not individual risk often times.

" I know God won't give me anything I can't handle, I just wish he didn't trust me so much."   -Mother Teresa

"The meaning of life is found in openness to being and being present in full awareness."   -Thomas Merton

"Be gentle with yourself."   -Max Ehmann

"Some people look at the world and say "why." Some people look at the world and say "why not?"   -George Bernard Shaw

"When one part of the body suffers, the entire body suffers with it."   -l Corinthians 12:26

"Cancer is a symptom of metabolic failure in the body that lets cancer grow."   -Author Unknown

6/16/04

Dear Auntie,

The call came and it's my darkest moment's fear. I have the big "BC" and I'm feeling numb all over. Lisa Starr gave me the results of my core biopsy pathology report on my left breast. I'm feeling like I'm in a grave yard of lost hopes seeing unwritten tombstones as I am running through the shadow of death. I feel like some of my many goals will never see the light of day. It's probably because I don't understand how I got it, ways to prevent it, what will happen and what my final prognosis will be. My fear is from the lack of knowledge I have about this illness. We have relatives that have died from cancer. I'm feeling overwhelmed because I have so many questions to this dance with death. This is not my "happy place." I think I need a lot of my family's love, support, and understanding during this very anxious time.

I read in a book that the *American Institute of Cancer Research (AICR)* said, "Each day our more than 10 trillion cells take 10,000 'hits' from agents that cause mutations. That's why it's so important to have strong, healthy bodies." They also

said "Sixty percent of all cancers in women and forty percent in all men are associated
with diet." In researching on their internet web site under expert report I found that
their group of experts feel cancer is preventable. Here's what they say, "The scientific
consensus is that cancers are largely preventable, and that the most effective means
of reducing risk are avoidance of tobacco use, consumption of appropriate diets, and
limiting exposure to occupational and other environmental carcinogens." I wonder
what all this is about. I'll have to do some more researching.

Someone once told me that breast cancer is determined by the level of estrogen,
length of exposure time, and all the factors involved in the cellular reproduction.
I don't understand what this all means.

Wow, the signs for breast cancer were all there---the lump I could feel, the enlarged
lymph gland under my left arm and the continual breast pain or burning.
Or is the burning my reflux problem acting up?

Terror and sadness fill me up as I think about the fact I have had such a great
professional career, wonderful life with my soul mate, and I have much more to
live for. I cried and I wept for endless hours mostly at night when Jim was sleeping.
I'm feeling like I'm in an empty desert without a cactus to break off for water and
the path out of the desert isn't visible. This is an emotional and physically draining
experience.

I know other women and men go through this, but why me? Why do people have
to go through this? I feel like I'm unraveling at the seams.

All I want to do is yell out, "Lord just get me through this. Help me to be strong
for myself and especially for my family." This is not the road I wanted to walk, nor
the mountain I wanted to climb. I wish I could see the struggle over and end to this
nightmare. Maybe then I will be all the wiser from it. This is not how I wanted to
spend my retirement years. I wanted to continue on with my doctorate degree thesis.
I'm worried even though I'm a seasoned, intelligent patient with previous cancer
experiences. Will I survive? I'm not so sure this time. I feel like the goldfish that

was just flushed down the toilet.

In reading an article I picked up, it stated in a chest x-ray we have a 1 in 350,000 chance of getting radiation due to the new x-ray films that are low dose radiation. It must be the same for mammograms. We are more at risk of getting radiation from other sources in our environment.

Help is needed. I'll call you.

Peggy

My lump is at the 3 o'clock position. Tumors are measured in cms. Attached is a tumor size chart as well as a pictures on how cells become cancerous, cells become cancerous from mutations, and how gene mutations occur.

I found on the internet from several sources that cancer cells are graded in how they are different from normal cells. Here's what I found:

Grades of Cancer Cells

Grade1-This is low grade or well differentiated cells. These are cells that appear normal and are not growing too fast. They are arranged in tubules when the pathologist looks at them.
Grade 2-These are moderately differentiated, intermediate or moderate grade cells. These cells could have characteristics between grade 1 and 3 tumors. The cells don't look normal and are faster growing than normal cells.
Grade 3-These are poorly differentiated cells or high grade cells. They don't look at all like normal cells and are very aggressive in their growth.

Pathologists and Their Jobs

The pathologist has the delicate job of looking at the cells to determine the grade, the kind of cancer, and the stage of the cancer. They often use the Scarff-Bloom Richardson grade system for the grading of the cells. The pathologist also looks at the necrosis or areas of cell death. Other important factors are the rate of cell division, the cells that have tubular structure formations, and the nuclear pleomorphism. The score the cells get is the grade. The pathologists have a difficult job because they have to determine the type of cancer and stage you have as well.

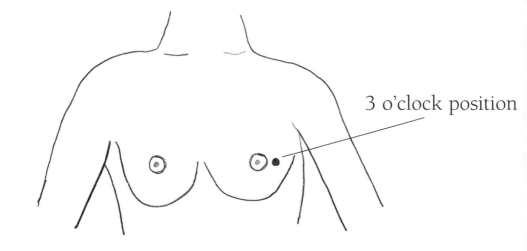

3 o'clock position

Tumor Sizes

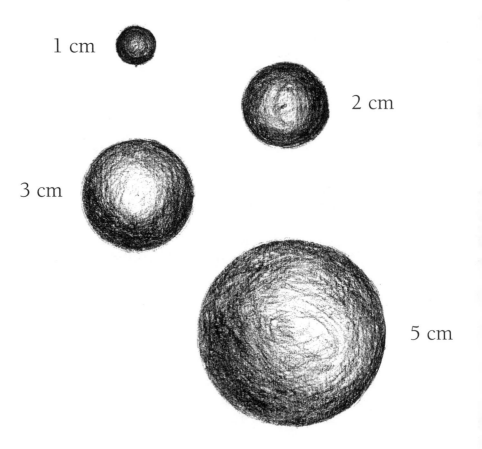

1 cm

2 cm

3 cm

5 cm

Two and one half centimeters (cm) = one inch.
One centimeter (cm) = 2mm.

How Cancer Cells Become Cancerous

Cancer Cells Have Irregular Shapes

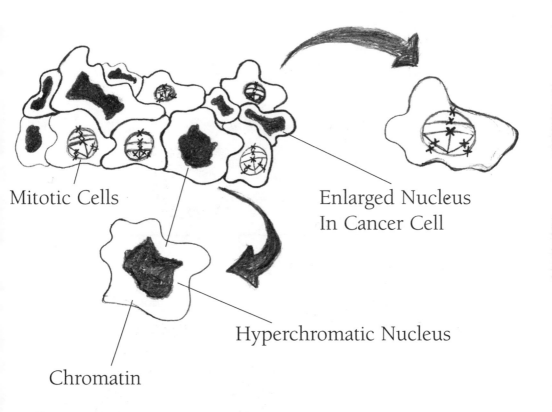

Mitotic Cells

Enlarged Nucleus
In Cancer Cell

Hyperchromatic Nucleus

Chromatin

How Cancer Cells Become Cancerous Masses

Normal Cells to Masses

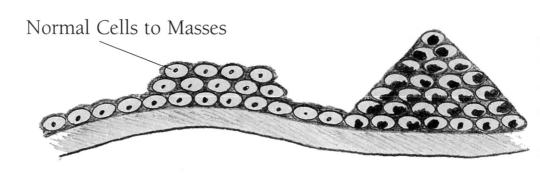

Mutated Genes Keep Copying

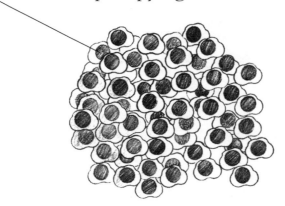

Basement Membrane

Epithethial Cell

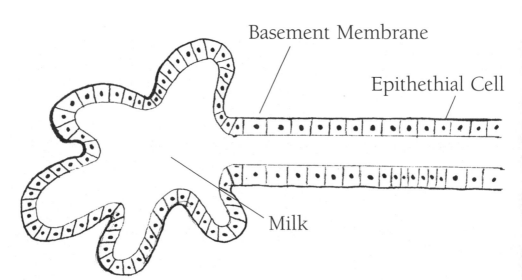

Milk

June 16,2004

Dear Peggy,

Today when you called and said you had been diagnosed with cancer, I felt so helpless--too far way to hug you or help you. My reassurance for you had to be on the phone and in my prayers. We both knew of this possibility, but to hear it called was very difficult.

My thoughts went back to my Mom and now this special granddaughter of hers. You who had given her such joy for her last seven years, now was facing the same disease that she had died from--breast cancer.

But that was fifty years ago, science and medicine has advanced. Today there are new options and treatments. Ask questions, continue to research and seek out the best medical advice. You must be the best advocate for your own health. If necessary to get an opinion ask, "What would you recommend if I was your daughter or wife?" and "Why?" before you make your decision on choice of treatment.

Above all, don't get discouraged. "All things are possible thru God." Remember in our journey of life we can't direct the wind, but we can adjust our sails. Be strong, take the challenge of beating this disease and keep the faith.

Love always,

Aunt Karen

P.S. Sharen called last night to check if I had heard what your diagnosis was and she said, " If it was me and it turned out to be cancer, I'd have both breasts removed and forget about any reconstructive surgery." They left early this morning for Washington, D.C. What a great place to take her teenagers to!

These procedures can save your life and your breast(s):

-A Breast Self Exam (BSE)

-A Clinical Breast Exam (CBE)
-Mammography
  Mammography picks up 90% of the DCIS cases and slow moving tumors.

Breast Cancer is the second leading cause of death in women.
Lung cancer is first leading cause of cancer in women. Breast cancer can be prevented if caught early.

Prognosis depends on the location and size of the tumors.

A **local occurence/reccurence** (in the breast) has a better long term prognosis.
Regional occurrence/reccurence (in the lymph glands) has a poorer prognosis. Cancer cells have gotten away from the primary tumor.
A **distant occurence/reccurence** (which has gone to the lungs, liver, spine or elsewhere in the body) has a lot poorer prognosis.

"A pessimist sees the difficulty in every opportunity, an optimist sees the opportunity in every difficulty."   -Sir Winston Churchill

"You gain strength, courage and confidence by every experience in which you really stop to look fear in the face. You must do the thing you think you can't do."
-Eleanor Roosevelt

"Fall down seven times, get up eight."   -Japanese Proverb

6/20/04

Dear Auntie,

Cancer must be called by it's name. This surely is every woman's very worse nightmare. I'm still feeling very powerless and helpless because I don't know where this road is going to take me. I feel like my life has scattered into a thousand puzzle pieces that won't go back together again. I just want this bad nightmare to end quickly.

I feel like I've stepped into a big black hole and I can't get up high enough to get out. There's such a sense of turmoil in me. I keep thinking, "I won't let this disease claim my life." I'm sure many other women have felt this way but I'm wondering, "Why me?" I don't want to get stuck here in this darkness. I want to get this over with, end breast cancer this year and go forward with my life. I'm a goal setter, so surely I can set goals to get over this. But then again there are so many unknowns, and I feel such a sense of urgency. Things I don't know, like how did I get this, and how can I prevent this from happening again? Can I be cured of this disease?

I'm sitting here like a limp rag doll body, having a bad day of grieving in my roller coaster ride of emotions. This has hit me in the face like a cold slap of winter. We all grieve in different ways and mine is summed up in three words: fear, sorrow and shock. At one moment I am wondering if I need to make preparations for my final departure. Then at another moment, I'm wondering why this happened and thinking how scared I am. I don't know that many people with breast cancer, so it can't be that common. Or is it something women don't talk about? Please give me some reasonable advice on how to deal with this.

I've been a faithful woman going for my mammograms each year including a clinical breast exam and yearly physicals. I have not been religious about checking my breasts. I've let myself fall apart physically by my gaining a lot of weight from my poor eating habits. Yet on two occasions, in 2001 and now in 2004, I found the lumps and went to my family doctor. I feel like a sword has stabbed me with grief. I'm wondering what is causing this life altering experience.

Call me soon. Hopefully I won't get stuck on the first chapter of pain. It seems like I'm trying to share my heavy burden. Yes, I am. My family is devastated by this news of the unknown. Bad day.

Peggy

June 25, 2004

Dear Peggy,

We've discussed on the phone several times how you must be your own advocate for your health.

This you have already started by requesting copies of all of your test results and I know you are very busy researching information on breast cancer. Here's another suggestion. Before your doctor appointments write out your questions that you want answered and bring that list with you. I usually start my list several days before an appointment, so I have a chance to add any new problems or questions that I come up with.

I always request my medical records to be informed of the results. To be your own advocate, we need to have a greater understanding and this can be done with our visual medical records.

The City of Hope, a Clinical Cancer Research Center Institute, has a great article enforcing the need to be our own advocate for our health. I'm enclosing it.

Don't get discouraged. This is a battle that you can and will overcome.

Love,

Aunt Karen

Today, cancer is the most treatable of all chronic diseases. Half of those diagnosed this year will live out their normal life span, while over 2 million living Americans are now considered cured of cancer. If you have cancer, here are some specific ideas for making your treatment a success.

1.Confront Your Fears

Cancer evokes powerful negative emotions: Fear that you are losing control over your body and your life. Anger that this is happening. Depression over what you must endure.

For people with cancer, these are all normal feelings. Suppressing them serves only to magnify them and will not help you to get better. The way to confront your fears is with education, understanding, faith, positive visualization and relaxation techniques.

Early on, connect with others who have been through the same experience (ask your doctor or hospital about patient support groups).

2.Take Charge

The leader of your treatment team is you. And the first rule with serious cancer is, get a second opinion. Your current doctor is usually happy to recommend someone, or you can research physicians whom you feel are experts in your cancer.

Take a close friend or relative along to consultations with you. Think in advance of questions you may want to ask, and have your companion take notes for review later (just advise the doctor beforehand). It's hard to deal with your emotions and absorb complex information at the same time.

3.Know Your Options

Learn as much as you can about your particular kind of cancer--become an expert. It sounds obvious, but try to find out what the latest and most effective treatments are before you commit to treatment. (Most physicians are reluctant to change a course of therapy once you've started.)

Centers designed by the National Cancer Institute share the latest information with each other nationwide and can generally offer the newest options and the most advanced treatments.

4.Fight Back

Keep asking questions throughout treatment and don't take anything for granted.

Make sure you have a doctor, a hospital and a treatment plan you feel confident in--don't just take someone else's recommendations on trust.

Don't worry about being a pest: experience shows that patients who aren't intimidated by their disease are the ones most likely to get better.

Don't think solely in terms of medical treatment. You may also need help with family, financial and spiritual issues.

Above all, don't lose your sense of humor. Every day, look for a little pleasure and enjoyment to offset the hours consumed by treatment.

City of Hope*

---

*The City of Hope has been treating people with cancer for 50 years and is a Clinical Cancer Research Center designated by the National Cancer Institute. We know cancer and will take the time to help you. If you or someone you know has been recently diagnosed, call 1-800-826-HOPE to find out more about treatment available at the City of Hope. For general information about cancer, contact their Cancer Connections hotline at 1-800-678-9990.

(Per 100,000 population)

Breast Cancer Is The Highest In:

North America-91.0
Western Europe-86.4
Northern Europe-84.4
Australia/New Zealand-67.4

Breast Cancer Is The Lowest In:
Southern Europe-41.4
Soviet Union-28.0
Japan-21.0

The Reasons could be diet, age of child bearing, life styles, and environmental exposures.

This is from: http://envirocancer.cornell.edu

Go to Cornell University of College of Veterinary Medicine-Facts Sheets-Program on Breast Cancer and Environmental Risk Factors.

"Blessed are those who mourn, for they shall be comforted."   -Mathew 5:4

"God will wipe away any tear."   -Revelation 7:17

"He who cannot rest cannot work; he who cannot let go cannot hold on."   -H.Fosdick

"Be strong and courageous. Do not be afraid or terrified…., for the Lord, your God goes with you; he will never leave you nor forsake you."   -Deuteronomy 31:6

6/29/04

Dear Auntie,

Thanks for talking to me the other night. I feel like my life has been turned upside down and I'm on a scary roller coaster ride which I hate doing. I am still wondering and wanting to shout out, "Why me?" Through this sleet and darkness I feel like my life is spinning out of control. I need to navigate myself out of bed, my safe haven. At night I cry when I'm alone. I don't want Jim to know how I feel. I'm extremely fatigued from lack of sleep.

You are lucky that you haven't had breast cancer with a mother who died from it. Maybe it was the daily aspirin, vitamin E or Fosomax that you take for your bones every day. Do you think cancer is skipping a generation?

The long waited for meeting on the sixteenth with Lisa Starr, the nurse practitioner involved with the breast department at the clinic finally came. She's an exuberant, eminently qualified physician's assistant. Lisa discussed this poorly defined, palpable area in my breast that shows up on an ultrasound. It doesn't show up well on my mammograms, as she showed us on the films. Dr. Hoyer had put a metal clip in during my biopsy to identify the location. Lisa showed us the information on the pathology report and we discussed different types of cancer, stages of cancer and treatment procedures. She told us about cancer options including surgery, lumpectomy, sentinel lymph node biopsy, axillary node dissections, a mastectomy, reconstruction, radiation, chemo and hormone therapy. Then we discussed a possible family history of breast cancer, genetic testing, previous cancer and further testing as the breast MRI. We discussed a radical video I had watched on breast cancer. She told us it isn't the standard of care in the United States. Lisa said my case would be presented at the cancer conference tomorrow for recommendations. I guess they do a case management approach to breast cancer which involves all the stake holders, or people involved in the treatment plan. When we left, Jim and I felt we understood cancer a lot more clearly before we bombarded the surgeon, Dr. Park Skinner, with our many questions.

Diagnosing breast cancer comes with many challenges. In the meantime I have been reading about diagnosing breast cancer from many sources. As I was reading, I came across one article about a study reported by the *New England Journal of Medicine* on six cancer centers in the Netherlands. I thought it was interesting because it said that MRI's found twice as many tumors as mammograms, but cost was an issue. Of 45 tumors on women, 32 were identified by MRI's whereas 22 were visible on mammograms. It went on to state in this article that mammograms missed 15-25 cases. It also stated MRI's were superior but had more false alarms. Then in another study on the internet by a *Breast Cancer Diagnosis* source on new approaches to MRI's, it said in a study one-third of breast abnormalities were found on MRI's than were present on x-ray mammograms. These abnormalities were found with women who had "dense" breasts on x-ray mammograms. Another study mentioned on the internet *WEB MD Health* talked about the value of MRI's in detecting additional tumors. Mammography detected 124 tumors (66%) while MRI's detected 152 (81%). The article goes on to state that more aggressive tumors can be missed by mammography. On the *Cancer Treatment Centers of America* web page (www.cancercenter.com) it tells a reader MRI's are useful in diagnosing breast cancer and finding the stages if you have dense breasts, implants, genetic predisposing, or previous cancer in a breast. So, since I have dense breasts I think I need an MRI to make sure some of the cancer isn't missed.

In researching the MRI's, I found there are advantages and disadvantages to a breast MRI. For example, the disadvantage is that it's expensive. If you are claustrophobic, it is a problem unless you go to an open scan. It's not a photo detecting device, doesn't pick up early signs of cancer as DCIS calcifications or microcalcifications, and the contrast dye goes quickly to the lymph nodes, so it might mean you don't have cancer. What are the advantages? An MRI can measure the blood flow to the tumor, the size, shape, and appearance of the tumor. It can show both breasts and the lymph nodes at the same time. The MRI is a useful in staging subsequent treatments, and it will show residual disease after cancer is removed. I learned that all tests have a purpose.

Today, we saw Dr. Park Skinner, a petite Asian doctor, for a surgical consultation. (Jim went along to provide an extra listening ear.) She diligently discussed different background information with us, including the two types of cancer I have and treatment options after doing a physical exam on me. Dr. Park Skinner discussed a modified radical mastectomy versus breast preservation therapy or a lumpectomy, axillary staging, followed by radiation. We also discussed chemotherapy depending on the size of my tumor and the auxiliary node status, as well as hormone receptors (estrogen/ progesterone),genetic testing, and HER2-Neu status. Staging seems to rely on the pathology report. The grade may be the same but staging for an individual can vary if you have a relapse at some point in your life. The grade can also change.

My surgeon, Dr. Park Skinner did talk to me about my long-term prognosis for breast conserving surgery, a lumpectomy. There is a slightly higher chance of getting a reccurrence back with breast preservation. We discussed a single mastectomy and a double mastectomy. She suggested I meet with a reconstructive doctor, in case we can't get clear margins from the invasive or infiltrating ductual cancer. We discussed genetic testing. I had many questions about the mammogram versus the ultrasound.

It's still a puzzle to me. I don't understand how I could have cancer, when I had an ultrasound a month earlier showing no cancer. My mammogram this time in 2004 barely showed any visible cancer by the metal clip. Because I have swelling under my arm, Dr. Park Skinner felt I should have a breast MRI which included my lymph glands. She warned me that this test isn't perfected and can have false positives. I felt more tests are better than fewer.

Jim and I were impressed with Dr. Skinner. She is knowledgeable, compassionate, honest, and yet optimistic as she laid all the cards on the table. Jim even stated as we walked out into the waiting room, "If I had breast cancer, I would want her to do it!"

This whole experience has been an acid layer of discovery. I have decided I want the lumpectomy procedure and it was scheduled. I want to try the least invasive procedure first and it will happen soon. Dr. Parker discussed problems with large breasted women and one breast. Or was that Lisa Starr? Each breast cancer victim has to make decisions, and some will decide differently. I realize we do not always have a choice. Some women don't want to worry, so they have one or both breasts removed. It's not like having your lymph nodes removed because you have cancer. This doesn't leave anyone with a choice. The swollen arm from the lymph nodes being removed is a matter of fact to many, as well as having one breast. The American Cancer Society tells us, "Unless cancer has spread to the skin, chest wall, and distant organs, long-term survival rates after a lumpectomy plus radiation therapy are similar to survival rates after modified radical mastectomy."

In 2001 when I discussed my earlier biopsy with my son, Chris, he told me, "It's not that unusual for some women to have their breast cut off. Women cut one breast off in this South American culture because they are hunters and shoot bow and arrows on that side." He wasn't sure if it was truth or myth. That made me feel a little better because I could pretend I was in South America.

I'm still wondering how this happened. I'm no stranger to cancer but, "Why me?" I read somewhere that overweight women with breast cancer are at higher risk to die from the disease. Also I read if you carry your weight around your waist like an apple, it's a bad sign. Now I am worried as I can't start a diet. On the internet it said a number of DCIS cases will turn into invasive cancer for some unknown reason.

Cancer can be caused from genetic causes as BRCA 1 and BRCA2, a family history of breast cancer, high breast tissue density, and biopsy confirmed hyperplasia, but especially atypical hyperplasia. I probably told you this before, but when cancer is diagnosed at the early stages there is a 95% survival rate for five years. So we women need to find tumors at an early stage while it is still curable. Sixty percent of the deaths do occur in women who are 65 years or older!

This is depressing me internally. I'm rocking and rolling in my bed at night as I can't sleep a wink. There can't be that many full moons either. Maybe my melatonin is low. I'm stuck on my nocturnal side in this merry-go-round of life as I go up and down. Kudos' to you for all that you do for me.

Love,

Peggy

Here's a few more cancer facts, terms, knowledge, concepts, pictures, and diagrams, pictures of types of breast cancer, lymph nodes locations, where they do the biopsies on lymph nodes, breast cancer stages, and some information on the signs of lymph node cancer and other data.

I searched the internet to find information on insomnia, which is a major problem for both of us. Enclosed is what I found. It maybe of some help.

1. Avoid caffeine products at least four hours before you go to bed. This includes coffee, cola, caffeine type teas and hot chocolate as these are diuretics. Besides caffeine products keep people awake. They say chamomile tea helps people to sleep but I've never tried it.

2. Take a warm bath and add calming mixtures which are sold in various stores to help you relax. This may be psychological.

3. Listen to soothing music and that means **no** TV before bed!

4. Biofeedback, meditation, prayer, yoga, reading, and thinking of peaceful thoughts can help a person to relax.

5. Don't eat supper late or snack before bedtime as your body will be too busy digesting, and you can get indigestion. I've read that warm milk, turkey, tuna, or bananas have tryptophan which is suppose to help you to sleep. Other foods you could eat which could be helpful include sweet corn, cherries, oats, rice, barley, ginger, and tomatoes.

6. Melatoin has been used in clinical trials to get patients to sleep. I read that vitamins B3 and B6 make melatonin. Foods rich in these vitamins would be good, I think.

7. Some people need proteins and complex carbohydrates before they go to sleep, so they don't wake up from a drop in blood sugar. I wonder if this would help Uncle Jim.

Treatment Choices, Further Diagnostic Options, Medical Findings, Prevention, Medical Terms

Cancer Facts, Terms, Knowledge, Concepts

Symptoms/Risks/Causes/Prevention:

Chemo Side Effects-Chemo has several side effects depending on the type, strength, and amount. They can include chemo brain (memory loss), lowered blood counts, fatigue, nausea, hair loss, and other menopausal symptoms.

Healing Problems-Problems can occur with healing if you smoke, have poor nutrition, or are diabetic.

Individual Risk Factor-This depends on the type of cancer, the size of the tumor and the number of lymph nodes involved, if the cancer has spread and if the cancer was positive or negative to hormones.

Prevention of Cancer- The American Cancer Society in their 2004 facts and figures states breast cancer can be prevented by: 1.avoiding obesity and weight gain 2.increasing physical activity and 3. minimizing alcohol. They go on to say, "Women should consider the increased risk of breast cancer associated with the use of combined estrogen and progestin hormone therapy in evaluating treatment options for menopausal symptoms."

(In American Cancer 2005 cancer facts and figures they state, "breastfeeding, moderate or vigorous physical activity and maintaining a healthy body weight are all associated with a lower risk of breast cancer." They also report "scientific evidence suggests that about one-third of the cancer deaths in the US each year are due to nutrition and physical activity factors, including excessive weight." It also states tobacco is a determinate for cancer risk.)

Breast cancer can be prevented by monthly breast self exams, clinical exams by your doctor, and mammograms. For women with dense breasts, a genetic breast cancer risk or a family history of breast cancer, it is wise to have ultrasounds and breast MRI's.

Diagnostic Procedures/Treatment:

Antitumor Antibiotics-These are antibiotics used to treat the tumors.

Aspirin-A drug that stops the production of hormones by reducing inflammation, when used daily. Some researchers feel it has a positive role in preventing breast cancer.

Axillary Lymph Nodes-These are the nodes under the arm, and they may need to be removed for accurate staging. The surgeon removes them from the bottom upward.

Claus Assessment Model-This is one of the two models used by doctors with Caucasian women to determine the chance of getting breast cancer. This is a good model for hereditary breast cancer. It's based on data from a large cancer and hormone study done in the 80's by the Center for Disease Control. The study determines the use of oral contraceptives, breast cancer, endometrial and ovarian cancer. It also considers 1st and 2nd degree relatives as well as their ages at the time of diagnosis.

Chemotherapy-Chemotherapy is drugs or medicines used to treat cancer that has metastasized from the original or primary tumor. There are more than 100 different drugs the oncologist can choose from. In some cases, chemo keeps the cancer from spreading, slows the cancer growth down, gets rid of the cancer completely in other distant sites, and can relieve some cancer symptoms.

Fluorscence Bronchoscopy-A blue light used to diagnose in situ.

Gail Model-A model based on the Breast Cancer Detection and Demonstration Project Data. The study assessed risk factors, breast screening, and development of breast cancer. The factors considered were first menstrual period, age at which you had a baby, the number of breast biopsies, and the number of first degree relatives with breast cancer. The model needs to be done on women under 20, minorities, and those who have had breast cancer for more data. It doesn't look at breast cancer history as far as ovarian cancers, breast cancers on the father's side or 2nd degree relatives with it. It does come with it's own set of faults. For example, it can over estimate women with breast biopsies, and under estimate women with inherited BRCA1 and BRCA2. It also can overestimate a women who had a mother or sister with breast cancer when older. This model predicts the risk of developing breast cancer over 5 years.

Genetic Mutation Tests-These tests measure inherited genetic mutations: BRCA1 and BRCA2. These cancers account for 5% of all cancer cases. BRCA1 is highly resistant to chemo. There are rogue tumor suppressor genes and when they are damaged a women is at risk for breast and ovarian cancer. If someone carries these genes in their family, they have a life time risk of 35-85%. Research shows a woman should have both breasts and ovaries removed for protection against this disease to reduce risk.

Grading and Staging-Tumors are graded and staged by a pathology report and various models are used to figure the risk factor from the results.

HER2/neu Positive-Women's tumors are tested for this, and if they are positive they can be put on Herceptin with standard chemo treatment.

High Risk Women-Women at high risk should have prophylactic mastectomy and oophorectomies. They should have clinical breast exams, chemo, prevention medications, mammograms, ultrasounds, and MRI's.

Hormone Therapy-This is when the patient is given hormones to block the estrogen in their body that is causing the cancer. Brand names include Tamoxifen (Nolvadex), Toremifene (Fareston) for pre and postmenopausal women that have receptor positive breast cancer. Megestrol Acetate (Megrace) is used for pre and postmenopausal women with metastases. Anastrozole (Armidex) is used for postmenopausal women only with receptor positive breast cancer that have metastases. Goserelin (Zoladex) is used with premenopausal women with breast cancer. Aromasin (Exemestane) and Femara (Letrozole) are used with postmenopausal women who have positive receptors and have breast cancer that has metastases.

Lumpectomy-This is the complete local removal of a tumor with clear margins. A patient often has radiation and takes hormone blocking drugs. Some patients would take chemo.

Mammograms-Mammograms use x-ray compression to get breast images by seeing the contrasts of breast tissue. The mammogram shows projected images, sees calcifications, but doesn't show aggressive cancer in very dense breasts.

Mastectomy-This is the surgical removal of a breast. This has been the standard of care in breast cancer treatment for many years.

Monoclonal Antibodies-These are used to block the protein receptors that are produced by breast cancer.

MRI'S(Magnetic Resonance Imaging)-This is a sensitive diagnostic tool that uses radio waves and strong magnetic fields by magnetic oscillation to identify abnormalities in the lymphatic system and diagnosis diseases by way of multi-slice pictures. These slices show up as the field lights. There is increased visualization where new blood vessels feed so the tumor shows up. The MRI does pick up masses, but can have false positive results as the mammogram. This is a more expensive procedure that often insurance companies won't pay for use as a diagnostic tool unless there is a good reason. (Some of the good reasons for MRI's could include inconclusive mammogram, a palpable abnormality with no mammography findings, distinguishing malignant from benign tumors or lesions, nipple discharge for no reason, additional tumors, recurrent breast cancer vs. scar tissue, cancer metastasis or the extent of cancer.) It's not a painful test because there is no compression. MRI's don't pick up calcifications and often doesn't pick up DCIS but it's very effective with women who have dense breasts, come from a predisposing family history of breast cancer, or have genetic breast cancer.

Other Useful Tools- These tools are Brachytherapy, ductual lavage, electrical impedance (T scan), flow cytometry (to detect rate of cell division), immunoassay (to detect antibodies) laser ablation, Miraluma breast imaging , nuclear medicine (scintimmography), optical density scan, optical imaging, Photodynamic therapy, positron x-ray (hair study) thermal imaging, and tumor markers. Some of these are in trials.

PET-(Position Emission Tomography)-This is an expensive test that involves accurate diagnosing of a tumor. It can detect different rates that cancer cells consume sugar or glucose as a substance is emitting a positron into your body. Cancer cells grow faster than normal, so a PET scan can detect them. This test is often used for metastic disease when they scan your whole body. Some feel it is not a real good test for breast cancer due to the false positives and poor spatial resolution. Others feel it is the best test because it can show whether cancer cells are active, not just there. It can tell if the tumor mass is active, growing, shrinking, and inactive. It has been used as a comparison tool to rule cancer out.

Sentinel Node Biopsy-This is a biopsy where they take the first lymph node out to see if the tumor has metasized. The doctor by standard policy will stop if this node is negative and not remove any further nodes. If there is a reason to suspect more cancer cells further down in the nodes the doctor will continue on. This is done by using a radioactive tracer injected around the tumor. The tracer travels to the cancerous cells, so that the surgeon can remove them for identification.

Steroid Hormones-These are high doses of progestogens used to reduce the tumor and the associated problems with the tumor.

Treatment Options for Breast Cancer:

1. Biopsy (tests for cancer)
2. Staging (what kind of cancer and how has it spread)
3. Treatment (any combo)

Lumpectomy-Removal of the tumor in the breast.

Radiation-Therapy with high energy x-rays on the cancerous area.

Mastectomy-Removal of the breast or breasts.

Chemo-Cocktails to destroy the cancer cells.

Hormonal-Hormone blocking drugs to stop the estrogen.

Medical Findings/Terminology:

Cancer-A disease which has cells that divide at a greater than normal rate and cause metastasis. Cancer is referred to as malignant tumor that undergoes some type of metastasis.

Carcinoma-This develops on the epithelia and endothelia tissue in the breast and skin. Metastasis can occur.

Estrogen/Progesterone Receptors-Patients have estrogen and progesterone receptors which can be treated by blocking them. Women with negative tumors are more likely to die from this disease than women who are estrogen positive.

Estrogen-A female sex hormone produced by the ovaries. It promotes menstruation, reproduction, and stimulates secondary sex characterizes. Estrogen can promote hormone dependent cancer.

Gene-A basic unit of heredity that is located on a chromosome in the nucleus of a cell.

Grading and Staging-Tumors are graded and staged on a pathology report. There are various models or scales that doctors use to figure the risk factors for the pathology report.

Types of Breast Cancer

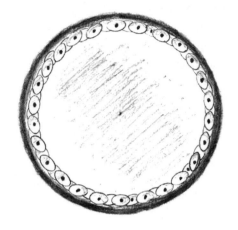

Normal Duct

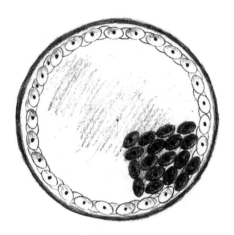

In Situ Cancer

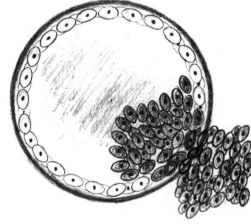

Invasive Cancer

Distribution of Axillary Lymph Nodes

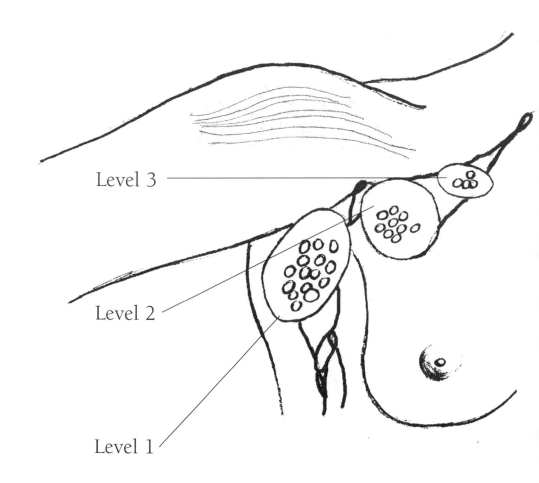

Biopsy

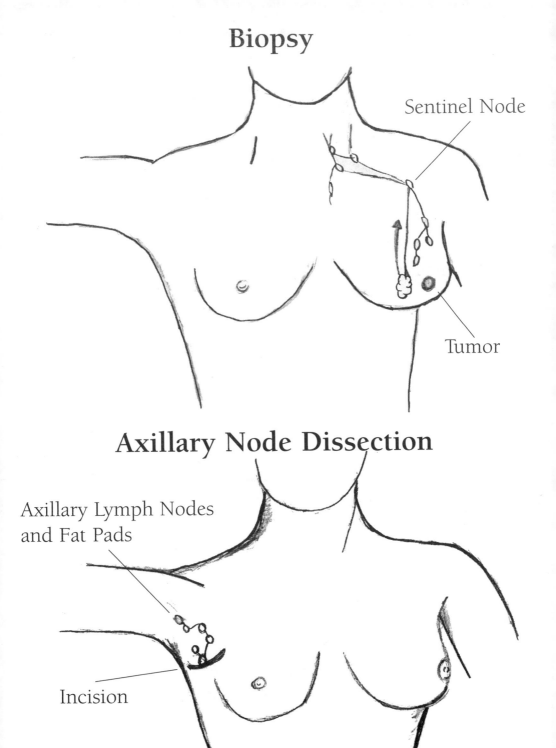

Sentinel Node

Tumor

Axillary Node Dissection

Axillary Lymph Nodes
and Fat Pads

Incision

Stages of Breast Cancer

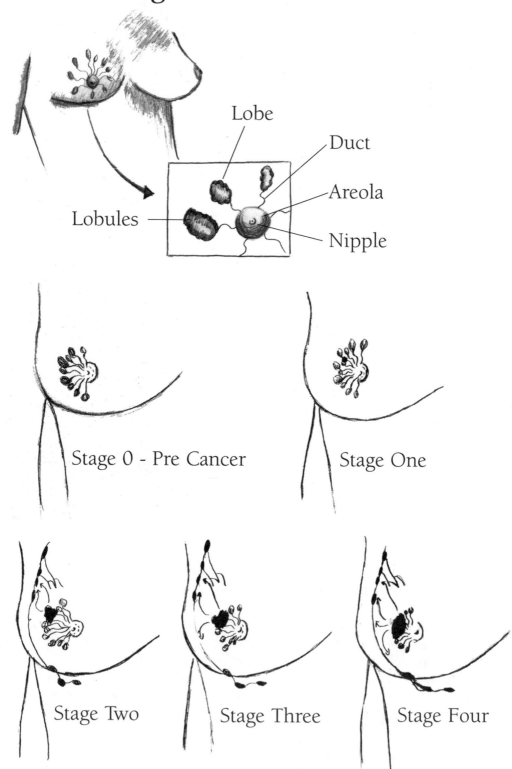

Lobe

Duct

Areola

Lobules

Nipple

Stage 0 - Pre Cancer

Stage One

Stage Two

Stage Three

Stage Four

The Signs of Lymph Node Cancer Include:
1. Enlarged node
2. Hard node
3. Bumpy node
4. Tender feeling node
5. You can't move the node; it's fixed and it doesn't change in size over the days.
6. It's been there for more than two weeks.
7. Several nodes could be connected.
8. The node can have an irregular shape.
9. You may have pain later, associated symptoms as weight loss, will not be eating, have fever or night sweats.

Symptoms of Non-Cancerous Lymph Nodes Include:
1. Moveable node
2. The node may be isolated but be clearly defined in its shape.
3. It can be infected, tender, or inflamed.
4. The node can feel like a pea or be enlarged.
5. It can change over different days.
6. The node may have a smooth texture.
7. It can feel soft.
8. The node can feel rubbery.

Lymph Node Survival Rates:

Lymph Nodes	Survival In 10 Years	Survival In 10 Years Without A Reccurence
No Cancer	80% plus	70% plus
1-3 Nodes	40-50%	25-40%
4-5 Nodes	25-40%	15-35%

Lymph Nodes Next To The Breast Area and Under The Arms:

Going From The Top Downward:
Axillary Lymph Nodes Level III: This is the area above the pectoralis muscle.
Axillary Lymph Nodes II: The are underneath the pectoralis muscle.
Axillary Lymph Nodes I: This is the area at the bottom level and at the lower end of the pectoralis muscle.

By The Neck:
The supraclavicular lymph nodes are located by the neck.

Inside The Breast:

These are the internal mammary lymph nodes.

Under The Breast:

The pectoralis major muscles and some of the axillary lymph nodes are located here.

Lymph Node Removal:

Lymph Nodes are removed from the bottom up in an axillary dissection. The sentinel node would be the exception.

Most Common Cancer Deaths in Women : From American Cancer 2004, "Cancer Facts and Figures"

1.Lung
2.Breast
3.Colorectal
4.Ovarian/Pancreatic
5.Non-Hodgkin's Lymphoma
6.Bladder
7.Melanoma (Skin)
8.Thyroid

"Cast your burden on the Lord and he will sustain you."   -Psalm 55:22

"Sorrow comes to all, and it often comes with bitter agony. Perfect relief is not possible except with time. You cannot now believe that you will ever feel the better. But....are sure to be happy again. Knowing this, truly believing it, will make you less miserable now."   -Abraham Lincoln

"I lift up my eyes to the hills-where does my help come from?
My help comes from the Lord, the maker of heaven and earth.
He will not let your foot slip-he who watches over you will not slumber;
Indeed he who watches over Israel will neither slumber nor sleep.
The Lord is your shade at your right hand;
The sun will not harm you by the day, nor the moon by the night.
The Lord will keep you from all harm-he will watch over your life;
The Lord will watch over you coming and going both now and forever more."
                    -Psalm 121

7/2/04

Dear Auntie,

Here's a few snapshots of what's been happening in Duluth, Minnesota. Today I went to see my family physician, Dr. Nisswandt, for my physical prior to my surgery. Hopefully, this will be my only surgery as Jim is a basket case over it. I had an EKG in February, so I only needed to have blood work done and a routine pre-operation physical. I've got the easy part. My doctor has to regurgitate my medical history on paper, before I can be approved for surgery. She needed to know all the medical problems of my genealogical family as well. Dr. Nisswandt went over my present prescriptions and what I should stop taking. We discussed my blood pressure going up recently and what to do in case of high readings. You know, I have started to develop " a little white coat syndrome." I have been approved for surgery and am a little worried. I haven't had surgery since I had a hysterectomy for cervical cancer in 1971. My biggest worry is being put totally under. I'm a somewhat healthy specimen for age 56 but with some health issues.

Once I made my decision to go for the lumpectomy in Dr. Park Skinner's office, I knew I would need to live with this decision. Life could change in a month. Later I went to see my family doctor, Dr. Nisswandt, and she assured me I could do this, and I'd be okay. She is an exceptional doctor that really understands where you are coming from and where you are going. I'm so glad we have such a conscientious family doctor. Dr. N. spends **a lot of time** talking with her patients. She eats real healthy, and I think she's vegetarian. Lisa and I have both seen her at the Whole Food COOP. We always think it's unusual we never see doctors out eating. Do they know something we don't know? They probably eat healthier than us!

I read somewhere that a healthy body weight can prevent cancer and other diseases. It went on to say excessive estrogen can set the stage for increased cell division and mutation. I have too much fat circulating in my blood, and my weight sure shows it. My triglycerides were 413 in 2003. That's way beyond the goal of 190. Added to this I have inflammation problems in my chest. I have to lose weight and I sure know it!

Oh, I forgot to tell you about my MRI results. It showed my breast cancer and a lymph gland area in the left side that needs to be looked at. I guess I have a simple cyst in my right breast and other cystic structures in both breasts. One can only put so much credence in this as the MRI can have false positives. Anyhow I haven't had problems with my right breast. By that I mean no lump, no pain, no discharge, no dimpling and all those other bad signs.

What is cancer? I searched through many sources to find out what cancer is. I found it to be a disruption in the delicate balance between cell growth and cell death. If there's too much cell division you have an increase in cell numbers or uncontrolled growth that isn't regulated with too little death of the cells. This is what causes cancer cells to develop. Think of it as an overgrowth of cells!

Cancer cells cluster and go to form cancerous tumors or masses because they want more of their gang. They anchor and adhere to their neighboring cells and tissues by way of receptors as appendages or legs as they attach to the healthy tissue pushing it out of the way, then go into the blood and the lymph vessels. They pile up like Humpty Dumpty on the wall but in layers like bricks. Normal cells want to be in order in a row, whereas cancer cells want to be in masses to infiltrate, invade and destroy tissue. Cancer cells want to be on the basement membrane of the lymphatic system by causing a mutation pileup. They are hyper triggers who want to control the growth and death of cells by metastasis.

A cell becomes a bad mutant boy when it's tired of it's everyday boring life. It's a gene that has an error or mistake. They get the nickname, "oncogenes." They don't want to exist in their present mundane state of existence. They busily make copies of themselves, so they become a whole gang to pursue anarchy like in the book *Animal Farm*. These bad boys refuse to cooperate and want a rumble war in your body. Cancer cells are free floating, disorganized, and have no filament bundles. They are always ready to be a gang, to hit and destroy good cells as they gang up on the chromosomes or DNA that effect cell growth. This is when they force the mutations to occur in the bases, phosphate groups, and the DNA molecules. Scientists have actually identified 100 oncogenes that take part in this cancer building process. Think of it like bees in a bee hive where everyone has a job!

The causes of cancer are what causes the mutations. These mutations happen every day in cells and are not all cancerous. The cancer cells have abnormal nuclei with abnormal amounts of chromosomes. These cells form mutations, gene amplifications, deletions, and duplications. For example, most of the time these mutations can be fought off by one's own body's immune system. We have a special police patrol that corrects these errors by shooting off special enzymes with their guns. These enzymes are protecting our DNA. Substances in our diet can effect DNA mutations as well. A lot of times the mutations are killed by this special policing force. The bad boys that are stronger survive and go on to be cancerous.

There are some "natural killer" cells, in fact an army of them, that fight cancer cells. We don't want anything to happen to this army in our body. That brings in our immune system which protects the invasion of organisms like bacteria, fungus and cancer cells. They send in these lymphocyte armies to fight the war. To fight the lymphocytes need trace minerals and vitamins. They get special strength from protein, need antioxidant nutrients and phyotochemicals to protect healthy cells from this invasion of free radicals. Antioxidants use a special substance they get from food to help the immune system fight this gang of bad boys. Phoytochemicals are found in the foods we eat, and they help to stop this mutant gang from committing more serious crimes. It's important to eat plenty of foods with vitamins A, E, and C. I think of Dr. Quillin's book, which I really enjoyed reading, and how he states a healthy body can better fight cancer. These chemicals can act as anti carcinogens along with the whole immune system to help in this cancer war.

Cancer surgery is necessary when cancer cells metastasis or anchor. This anchoring causes them to grow fast or slow. Surgery, radiation, chemo and hormone therapy are necessary to stop them in their tracks. Cancer can kill fast or slowly.

I'm starting to feel nervous about surgery. I'm on this rocky road, I don't know the way and I don't know what's at the end of the road. This is a very scary experience. I'm brave and optimistic on the outside, but scared on the inside. The shades of my eyes want to close. Maybe, I'll cry myself silly.

Jim says I'm getting absent minded, becoming a poor manager of time and he's noticed my attention span is shorter. I'm wondering if it is the Efflexor pills I'm on. I feel like I'm in the movie," Sleepless in Seattle." At night I am awake due to severe hot flashes and I turn all around in bed. I told Jim I wanted the headboard turned north and he said, "You know, that's crazy!" Sometimes I get up and go on the computer. I write to Karla (my Blue Cross-Blue Shield case manager), Linda, Wendy, Helen, Kay, and others.

This sounds sounds like a sad song that I didn't want to sing, but my stress shrouds the enormity of what I feel. I just can't stop the pictures in my mind and I wonder if I should plan my funeral, complete a living will, write my obituary, so Jim won't be stressed, clean or organize my house. Then again, I think I'm not going to let cancer take me and I can beat this.

I read on the internet that breast reduction can prevent the risk of breast cancer in women who are at high risk. It reduces the density somewhat but there's no guarantee in this procedure.

How are you feeling? Congratulations on becoming a grandmother of twin boys! I hope Shannon, Max, and Sam are doing fine.

Love,

Peggy

Here's what an MRI looks like, in case you have to have one someday, a picture of ductual in situ cancer, some more cancer knowledge, types of breast cancer, hereditary and genetic breast cancer percentages. I find it interesting that 80% of the women have no family history of breast cancer. I wonder what causes breast cancer for these women.

Breast Cancer Occurrences:

No Family History of Breast Cancer-80% (I've seen 70-90% as well.)
Hereditary Breast Cancer-5% (I've seen 5-10%.)
Some Family History of Breast Cancer-15%

Types of Breast Cancer and Occurrences:

Invasive Ductual-65% of the cases (I've seen this percentage even higher.)
Invasive Lobular-19-15% of the cases
DCIS-10-15% (I've seen this percentage even a lot higher.)
Tubular-6-8% of the cases
Colloid-2-4% of the cases
Mudullary-2-4% of the cases
Other-2-4% of the cases

72

Duct and Lobe Cancer:

According to American Cancer…
80% of breast cancer is in the ducts
20% of breast cancer is in the lobes

If You Have Genetic Breast Cancer:

Hereditary-7%
Familial-22%
Sporadic-71%
Total: 100%

Hereditary Breast Cancer:

BRCA1-30%
BRCA2-15%
Unknown Hereditary Types-55%
Total: 100%

Before Surgery, Types of Surgery Procedures, Cancer Types

Cancer Facts, Terms, Knowledge, Concepts

Symptoms/Terminology/Findings:

Annalgesic Drugs-These drugs can promote metastsis. They can impair the immune system which needs to be strong after surgery to fight tumors and cancerous cells. Tramadol is better than morphine as it doesn't suppress the immune system. It stimulates the natural killer cells. Morphine stimulates angiogenesis and apoptosis in four Life Extension studies. Avoid morphine and opiates if you can, and use other drugs that don't depress the immune system.

Anaplasia-A benign tumor that is disorganized but encapsulated in a mass that doesn't invade the tissue.

Angiogenesis-The formation or genesis for new blood vessels with nutrients and oxygen to support the cancerous tumor mass.

Apotosis-Cell death that is programmed.

Breast Cancer As A Symptom-Six percent of the women have breast cancer as a symptom, so it's rarely found by the typical women according to some sources.

Cancerous Lump-A cancerous lump underneath the skin feels hard like a rock with irregular edges.

Carcinogenesis-This is what the bad boys are called when they become cancer anarchists.

Carcinoma in Situ-This is a precancerous condition where the cells may not spread to the surrounding tissue. It is in one place unless invasion occurs.

Comedo Non-Invasive Cancer-A type that has "necrosis," which is dead cancer cells. It's fast growing and the cells die from a low blood supply.

Cribiform Non-Invasive Cancer- A type of non-invasive cancer with holes between the groups of cancer cells. Some think it looks like Swiss cheese.

Distal-This is when the pathologist looks at the nodes farthest from the chest wall.

DNA (Deoxyribonucleic Acid)-This is a substance found in human cells to reproduce chromosomes and viruses. It contains all the genetic information needed to reproduce another functioning cell.

Estrogen Receptor (ER)-A protein, receptor molecule is where the estrogen will attach.

Estrogen Receptor Assay (ERA)-This is a test done to see if a cancerous tumor is hormone dependent and can be treated with hormonal therapy. There's also a progesterone receptor assay.

Extracellular Maxtrix-Cancer cells can dissolve this with their matrix and make tunnels in the tissue.

Extensive Intraductal Component-This is cancer cells throughout the length of the duct.

Her-2/neu (Human Epidermal Growth Factor Receptor 2)-An oncoprotein that resides on the cells surface and promotes growth. In about 30% of breast cancer cells there is an excessive amount of growth and the cancer can be 25% more aggressive. This is also a name for the gene on the cell surface protein. This gene can amplify by making extra copies of itself in it's nucleus.

Invading Cancer (Infiltrating, Invasive)-Cancer that spreads past its site of origin.

Li Fraumeni Syndrome-This is what some individuals inherit. It's one functional gene from a parent who is predisposed to cancer.

Luteal Phase Surgery-The later part of your menstrual cycle when you could have surgery.

Mass Growth-It may take several years for a tumor to grow, so that you can feel it.

Malignant Tumors-These are usually distant tumors that are either carcinomas or sarcomas.

Metastasis-Occurs when tumors move their cancer cells to a new place or organ.

Multicentric Disease-This is cancer that is in two or more areas.

Neoplasm-Another name for a tumor.

Obesity-Two-thirds of the women who are premenopausal that have breast cancer are obese.

Occult DCIS-A pathologist can only find this as he looks at the breast tissue.

Oncology-The study of neoplasia.

Oophorectomy-Removal of the ovaries as a preventative measure in reducing estrogen production.

P53 Gene-This is the tumor suppressor gene and DNA guardian that starts the repair when a mutation occurs. If you inherit this gene on chromosome 17, you are predisposed to cancer and can get Li Fraumeni's Syndrome.

Papillary Non-Invasive Cancer-This is a type of cancer that grows with fingerlike projections toward the inside of the duct.

Phantom Breast-When the patient misses her breast.

Proximal-The pathologist looks at the nodes in order from the closest to the farthest from the chest wall.

Seroma-Fluid in the surgical cavity.

Solid Non-invasive Cancer-A wall-to-wall cell growth of non-invasive cancer.

Specimen -The tissue removed.

Supraclavicular Nodes-These are nodes around the collar.

Surgery Induced Immune Suppression-This can happen from treatments and some people use melatonin, lactoferrin, Echinacea, MGN3 to enhance cellular activity according to Cancer Adjunct therapy protocol Life Extension, (four studies).

Tumor Growth-Breast cancer tumors that are slow moving usually take one hundred days to grow. It takes three months for a cell to divide into two.

Types of Cancer-Invasive, Carcinoma in Situ (ductual and lobular), Non-invasive Cancers (Solid, Cribform, Papillary, Comedo).

Diagnostic/Medical Procedures:

Axillary Dissection-The removal of the nodes under the arm in three areas, levels I, II and maybe III.

Drain-This is a bulb shaped device that attaches to the skin, so it can drain the fluid through a tiny incision. It is held in place with a single stitch, and it can be very irritating as it heals.

Level I-The lowest point or bottom level, below the lower edge of the pectoralis major muscle. It is the uneven line of the axillary system.

Level II-This lies underneath the pectoralis major muscle and is the midway line in the axillary system.

Level III-The highest point above the pectoralis minor muscle. It's unusual for cancer to skip Nodes I and II and to have cancer in III. The surgeon often removes fat pads with the 10-20 nodes in Levels I and II to prevent lymphedema.

Lumpectomy-A simple procedure that removes the whole lump, while conserving as much of the breast tissue as possible.

Lymphedema-A condition that involves swelling, can be painful and disabling in the arm or leg. It's from having lymph nodes removed.

Lymph Nodes Adjacent to the Breast Area-There are lymph nodes in five areas adjacent or near to the breast. They are supraclavicular lymph nodes, axillary nodes level III, axillary nodes II, axillary nodes I from the collar bone going downward. There are also internal mammary lymph nodes on the inside borders of the breast.

Mastectomy-A surgical procedure where the entire breast is removed.

Modified Radical Mastectomy-This is when the muscles of the chest wall are spared. This is the procedure most women have if they have lymph nodes involvement.

Negative Lymph Nodes-These are nodes that don't show malignancy.

Negative Margins-Negative margins are clear of cancer.

Non-skin Sparing Mastectomy-This is a procedure that allows you to wear a breast form.

Partial Mastectomy-The lump is removed and a certain margin of the tissue. The procedure could involve a wide local excision, segmental mastectomy, partial mastectomy, quadrantectomy or a tylectomy.

Positive Lymph Nodes-Nodes that show malignancy.

Positive Margins-These are margins that contain malignant tissue.

Radical Mastectomy-A procedure when the entire breast, the lymph nodes in the armpit, the major pectoral muscles, and all lymph nodes in the chest wall are removed to improve chances of surviving. You can still get lymphedema.

Sentinel Node Dissection-This is the first node area.

Simple (Total Mastectomy)-The lymph nodes are removed as well as the entire breast if you have invasive and in situ cancer.

Skin-sparing Mastectomy-This is where skin from the stomach is used to make a breast.

Standard Axillary Dissection-Involves removing 10-25 nodes.

Treating Hot Flashes-Patients will be advised to deal with hot flashes in any of the

76

following ways: use antidepressants, avoid spicy foods, avoid stress, avoid toxic people and environments, use black cohosh, cut down on hot liquids as coffee and tea, dress in layers, drink chamomile tea, have a fan by your bedside, carry a mini fan in your purse for emergencies, listen to relaxing music, have a positive attitude, do relaxation exercises as mediation and imagery, pray, have water by your bedside or a wash cloth, walk, take vitamin E, and do visualization exercises. Always ask your doctor about taking herbal drugs and vitamin supplements first.

Medical Team Members:

Mammogram Technologist-A person who reads the mammograms.

Medical Oncologist-The doctor who specializes in chemo, hormone therapy and other cancer drugs.

Pathologist-A doctor that examines your cancerous tissue and other fluid samples. The pathologist also tests for protein and hormone receptors.

Plastic Surgeon-The doctor who performs reconstruction after a mastectomy as well as plastic surgery.

Other Oncology Personnel-This could include nurses, social workers, dieticians, physical therapists, a psychiatrist, counselors, mammogram technicians, nurse practioner, and spiritual clergy.

Radiation Oncologist-The doctor who uses radiation treatments on the patient for cancer.

Radiologist-A doctor who uses radiation treatments on the patient for cancer.

Skilled Medical Team-A team of doctors that are qualified and can consult with a patient on cancer information, procedures to be done, based on research and expertise.

Surgical Oncologist-The doctor that specializes in cancer surgery.

Who Will Get Breast Cancer?

Twenty to thirty percent of women will get breast cancer due to their age, family history, early menstruation, late menopause, not giving birth, not giving birth until after 30 years of age, never having breast fed, the use of oral contraceptives, long term use of HTR (hormone replacement therapy), history of endometrial cancer, family genetic history BRCA1 or BRCA2 cancer or other rare cancers, Jewish heritage, or high socioeconomic status.

Seventy to eighty percent of women will get breast cancer from life style choices as diet, alcohol (2% roughly), large body mass. or obesity, emotional, social issues and exposure to toxins.

Breast MRI

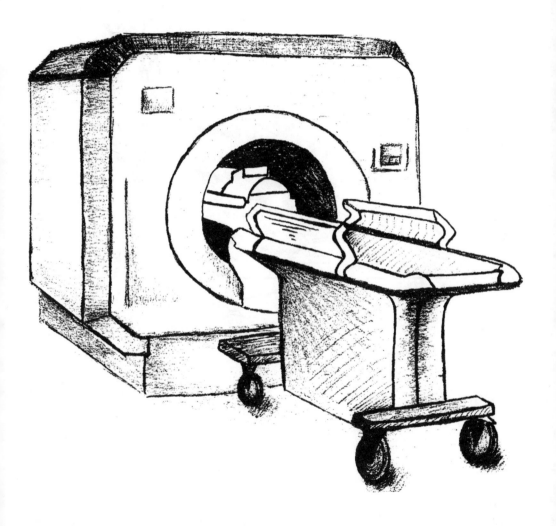

Ductual Carcinoma In Situ

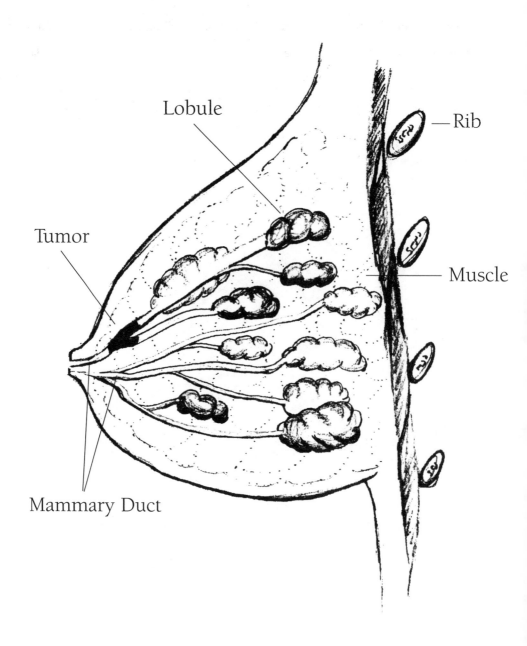

Lobule

Rib

Tumor

Muscle

Mammary Duct

July 2, 2005

Dear Peggy,

Today I spent a lot of my time reading over your letters and all the information you have sent me about breast cancer. I am so pleased you are keeping me up-to-date. My worries are greater when I don't know what's happening.

All of these medical appointments, various tests and the big decisions you have to make in such a short time are tough. Decisions and choices are always hard, even more so when it is your life. The "What ifs?" and "Should I?" or "How can I do this?" must go around and around in your mind. Remember to always ask for God's guidance through all this. He's never let me down and he won't you either. You are always in my prayers.

I am so pleased that Jim has put his summer plans on hold to be with you all the way in your fight to beat breast cancer. Together as a team with good medical help you will conquer this disease. His all out support for you must be very comforting. Give him a special hug from me for being such a great guy!

This week we will be celebrating the freedom of our country. As those sky rockets shoot off, I hope you will remember that soon you will be able to celebrate your freedom from breast cancer.

Take care dear Peggy and always remember how you are loved by so many.

Love always,

Aunt Karen

The internet tells us…..
-younger women
-older women
-some men (1%)
-Caucasian women who don't seek treatment early enough.
-African American women who don't seek treatment early enough. (They have a higher fatality rate.)
-Some Native American women who have a lower incident rate from not seeking treatment early enough. (They have a higher fatality rate in these cases.)
-Some Jewish women due to race and genetics.
-Those with genetic breast cancer.

How Can We Prevent Cancer Deaths?

1. We should make healthy life style choices as not drinking or smoking.
2. Regular daily exercise is important because it reduces a woman's risk by 33-55%.
3. Maintain normal body mass or weight for regulate estrogen levels.
4. Good emotional health or inner peace is vital to the immune system.
5. Know your family cancer and breast cancer history. Be sure to tell your doctor if you have a strong family history of breast cancer with two or more first degree relatives who have had breast cancer.
6. Find out if your breasts are dense from ultrasounds and mammograms.
7. Watch environmental toxins and make safe choices in your daily living.
8. Eat a healthy plant based diet with lots of fruits, vegetables, grains, low fat foods, more fish, organic beef (or low fat choices), organic chicken (or hormone free), and organic calcium choices (or low fat choices). If you are tumor estrogen positive watch the excessive phytoestrogen choices until more research studies are completed.
9. Tell your doctor if you have had high doses or radiation to your chest wall in the past, have had lobular carcinoma in situ, atypical hyperplasia or previous biopsies.
10. Let your doctor know if you have had ionizing radiation as a child or at other crucial time periods in your life.

"Grief can heal anything with time."   -Peggy Anderson

"God doesn't play dice."   -Albert Einstein

"The Lord made everything for a purpose."   -Proverbs 16:4

"He will never give us a burden greater than we can handle."   -Corinthians 10:13

7/8/04

Dear Auntie,

Yesterday I had breast cancer surgery at St. Mary's Hospital. I had to stay one night in the surgical recovery part of the hospital. They had trouble getting the breathing tube down my throat. I didn't know before that I have a constricted airway. Consequently, they had to give me a lot of morphine for pain as I couldn't swallow the pills and I kept throwing up. Lisa Starr and Dr. Park Skinner came to see me. Jim brought me two stuffed puppies that he put on my chest. I'm not sure if he meant it for me missing my puppies (Smokey Joe and Peanut Butter) at home or because I might lose my own puppies at some point. My kids, Lisa and Chris, came along with Joel. I felt dilapidated. Breast cancer surely is a family experience.

Last night someone died after surgery in intensive care recovery. It was hard to sleep because the family was outside my curtain type room. This was a very mournful experience for all involved. A minister was there counseling the family. I never thought about dying after surgery as all my worries had been about surgery. It sort of reminded me of the book I use to read with my students called, *Tuesday With Morrie*. Death is inevitable for us all.

According to Jim, I had a left breast lumpectomy, sentinel node biopsy, and axillary node dissection. I had twenty-one nodes removed under my left arm. Of the twenty-one nodes, there was one that was cancerous and positive for metastasis adencarcinoma. A drain had to be placed for lymph node drainage and emptied several times a day. I think I will be able to do this myself and record the amount of fluid.

Thank goodness, I had that breast MRI. It picked up this metastic tumor and surrounding tissue under my arm in the axillary area. Hopefully, all the breast cancer is removed. I still think about the fact that MRI's are not the standard of care because of the cost to insurance companies. Women's lives are more important. We need to have more diagnostic equipment available as part of the standard of care in Duluth, MN. Women need the right tests or machines to diagnose and treat breast cancer!

Today we are at the *Inn by The Lake*, a hotel at Canal Park, with my Hydrocodone pain pills and super-sized chest bandage. Hydrocodone has become my best friend for the moment and I will try to get off these as soon as possible. I know when I lay down to not move off of my back, as I'm afraid that my chest will rip open. Maybe that's a figment of my imagination at work. Last night I screamed out unconsciously in pain. I screamed so loud that it even woke me up!

Jim is working for the *Edgewater* and they own the *Inn By The Lake*. We are getting a special employee discount to stay here along with medical reasons. Chris, Lisa, and Jim are checking on me. Our wood floors are being done in our house, and I can't be at home because of my asthma. There's no way to get to the third floor to sleep.

The room here is a suite and it's really nice with a well supplied refrigerator and has a very nice living room. They have a great continental breakfast each morning and tonight we can even make smores on an open pit. The view of Lake Superior is so refreshing. I feel like I'm in Nantucket or Martha's Vineyard again. Tonight we have to move to a different room but one that has a deck, and we'll be just a hop, skip, and jump to the lake walk. It's a scheduling issue but we can't be choosey because they will move our bags and the biggest piece of baggage, namely me. I'm so impressed with the accommodations and care they give their guests. I'll have to write them a note besides personally thanking them.

This is all I can write. I'm having trouble focusing due to the Hydrocodone pain pills I'm on. I was put on Efflexor prior to surgery for hot flashes but it is also a antidepressant. I felt I had to go off of it before surgery.

I feel rough around the edges, so I am going back to bed. I'm just hoping all the cancer is gone. Right now I feel like a human drain without a plug. I'm feeling like someone should throw me a life line. Going through cancer has made me value life more than ever. It is such a complex process going through cancer. It's a balancing act of sorts. My Lisa is going to come over soon as I'm feeling ill. Oh, here's a few surgical pictures I added later to help you understand the procedures and choices of breast conserving surgery.

Peggy

Types of Incisional Surgery

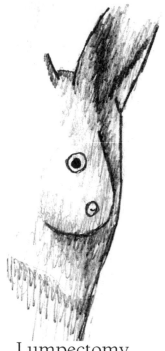

Lumpectomy

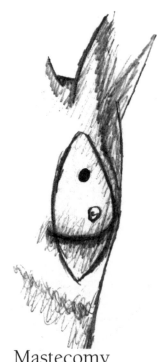

Wide Excision

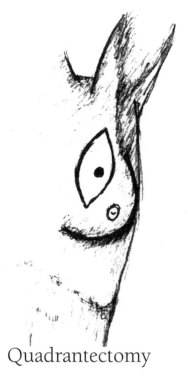

Quadrantectomy

Mastecomy

A lumpectomy removes a lump from the breast. This may include lymph node removal.

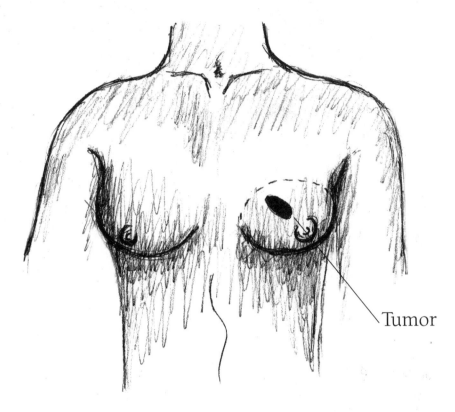

Tumor

Tumor removed and surrounding tissue

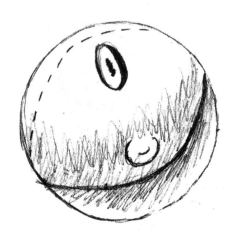
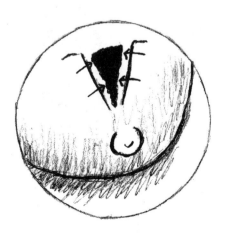

Stages of The Breast Tumors

0-There may be cancerous cells in the duct or lobules. This stage is noninvasive and the lymph nodes are not involved. These cases most often involve DCIS, LCIS and Paget's disease.

1 (I)-The tumor is no more than 2 centimeters. There is no lymph node involvement, so it is noninvasive.

2 (II)-The tumor is smaller than 2 centimeters or could be larger than 5 centimeters. There may be regional lymph gland involvement.

3 (III)-The tumor is larger than 5 centimeters, there may be spread to multiple axillary nodes with invasiveness into tissue and other nodes. The breast bone and collar bone may also be involved. Stage 3 is considered advanced node development.

4 (IV)-This is distant spread to other body organs and the skin. It may or may not have spread to the lymph nodes.

In Summary:

T=Tumor (local disease)   Tumors are staged Tis or O, T1, T2, T3, T4
N=Nodes (regional disease)   Nodes are staged NX, N0, N1, N2, N3
M=Metastases (distant disease)   Metastases is staged M0, M1

Tools often used to index tumor involvement: Van Nuys Prognostic Index (VNPI)

Stages of Lymph Node Tumors:

N1-The cancer has spread to axillary nodes and is moveable.
N2-The breast cancer has spread to axillary nodes and it is fixed.
N3-The cancer is spread to the internal mammary nodes.
Nx-This means that node involvement isn't determined.
No-This means there is no node involvement.

Stages of Metastases Involvement:

M0-No distant spread to the organs
M1-There is distant spread to the organs as the lung, liver, brain, bone, lymph nodes over the collarbone.

July 7, 2004

Dear Peggy,

Hallelujah! I was so thankful when Jim called and told me the surgery was over.

As you know, I am a strong believer in the power of prayer, so last night and this morning until Jim called, I've been busy offering up many prayers for you and for God to guide your surgeon.

The word surgery always seems to give us a chill. The thought "what if something goes wrong" creeps in. It is so important to have a good medical team.

Today must be a very painful day for you, so here's a smile for you. Before Sharen and her family left for vacation, I sent the kids some extra "pocket money" for souvenirs and asked them to send me a letter when they got home about what impressed them the most of all the wonderful sights in Washington, D. C., my all time favorite city. Here's what Landon wrote:

"Dear Grandma,

My trip was fun. We went to see big monuments. I also saw memorials. We went to the Mall too. My favorite part was swimming at the hotel. Thank you for the money. What I bought was a shot glass at the Capitol.

Love,

Landon

Landon soon turns thirteen. No letter was received from Emily, but on the phone she told me she liked "everything!" She bought a T-shirt and a spoon for her collection. She also has a birthday this month and will be sixteen.

Jim enjoyed the pictures Sharen sent us of the new World War II memorial. He was stationed in the South Pacific for 37 months with the Air Force during that war.

My all time favorite travel destination is D.C. All those memorials and monuments I find awesome. The Smithsonian buildings on the Mall are so full of history. If my health ever allows me another trip, I would go back there.

Peggy, I hope and pray that today's surgery was a complete success and all the cancer is gone. Take good care of yourself, take it easy and give yourself time to heal. Please call me as soon as you as up to it.

Today we have much to give thanks for--your surgery is over.

Love always,

Aunt Karen

"It takes two to speak the truth--and so speak and another to hear!" -Thoreau

"Rest in the Lord and wait patiently for Him." -Psalm 37:7

"I will give peace…and none shall make you afraid." -Leviticus 26:6

"He leadeth me beside still waters. He restoreth my soul." -Psalm 23:2-3

"Do not let your hearts be troubled and do not be afraid." -John 14:27

7/13/04

Dear Auntie,

Follow up appointments are important to my breast cancer treatment. I went to see Dr. Park Skinner today for a follow-up visit. She discussed with me the findings of my surgery from the surgical pathology report. Dr. Skinner explained that my additional axillary node did show metastases with the lymph node almost completely replaced by a tumor which may have accounted for the reason it didn't take up the radioactive blue dye. A partially blue breast! (Now that would make an interesting card!) Thank God, I had a breast MRI. Lymph nodes are the way cancer spreads in the blood stream. (Some can escape and grow elsewhere in the body for years by no fault of the doctor.) Typically surgeons would stop at the sentinel node biopsy, but my axiliary node farther down showed something on the MRI!

My breast cancer shows infiltrating ductual carcinoma grade 2 out of 3, as well as extensive ductual carinoma in situ. That means I have two types of cancer. The cancer has spread in my breast to lateral, inferior, and medial margins. The tumor in the breast was 1.5 and under the arm it was 2.5. If you include the extensions it is higher. Oh, I read on the internet some interesting information from the M.D. Anderson Center in Houston. It stated that a women's risk of breast cancer death increases by 10% with each additional tumor length. Maybe that's why you have to go by the final pathology report which can change with more tests and surgeries in this area.

My family members, Jim and Lisa went with me to this appointment. I took both of them upon their insistence. Lisa almost passed out due to the heat and her weak stomach for this type of news. In our family, Chris, when he needed stitches would sit up and pretend to be the doctor as he was having his knee stitched two times. Well, Lisa is the opposite. She's the loud one screaming in the other room. Lisa ended as the patient at one point during my office visit. She was passing out from the heat, looking at my stitches and the draining tube. The lesson is, "Don't take weak stomach relatives with you!" I told Lisa that the next time she should stay home and let me explain it to her.

My doctor discussed my medical pathology report. There's the part about estrogen and progesterone receptors. My tumors are positive for estrogen and progesterone, so my breast cancer can be treated with hormone blockers. (Being off hormones is a real killer. I didn't know I'd miss them so much. The hot flashes are not just bad, they are really bad!) The test for my tumor showed I had HER-2/neu with a score of 2 plus. I guess a FISH test (a test to find extra copies of the HER2/neu gene) may be done at some point.

Dr. Park Skinner told me that I didn't need anymore surgery on my lymph node. She said that I would need chemotherapy, radiation, or hormone therapy. Chemo is not something that I want to do, just like I don't want to lose my breast. The doctor told me that three out of five margins still continue to have tumor in the lateral, inferior, and medical margins. She discussed with me again the option of a mastectomy and re-excision to free myself of the cancer. Dr. Park Skinner said she could try for clear margins and I opted for this. I couldn't see myself with one large breast. We also discussed a mastectomy with reconstruction. I said I would pursue this option, in case it was necessary, by meeting with Northland Plastic and Reconstructive Surgery.

My mind is playing a replay or rewind on doing this again. But, I decided to have a re-excision to try to get the margins clear. It is scheduled for 7/15/04. This time I will be having a local anesthesia with sedation, so I won't be having any difficulties with a breathing tube. Last time they told me if I ever were to have a breathing tube again, I would need a scope. I couldn't swallow for up to nearly 24 hours. The restriction could be from gastric reflux problems.

How are you feeling and what have you been doing? I'm worried that I am plaguing you with way too much. Maybe this is a typical of overly involved cancer patient trying to get out of the black hole. As a cancer patient, I just can't find the first step up.

You know, when I was painting so excessively in the living room, hallway and dining room, I had two bad chest cramps. My sister-in-law told me that I should stop and continue what I was doing at another time. She was concerned that I was over extending my muscles, ligaments and tissues in that area. Now I am wondering if this is when some of the cancer moved to under my arm. I guess we'll never know, but maybe I should of listened to her wisdom.

You asked me on the phone when I said, "Why me?" You said, "Why not you? You will find a way to learn from this experience to teach others about this disease." I'm not at all feeling that way now.

Lots of love,

Peggy

Tumors

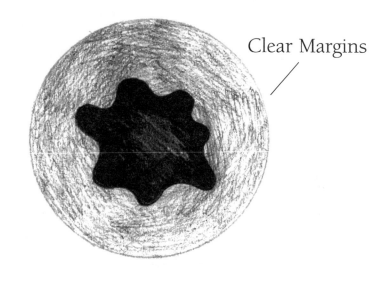

Clear Margins

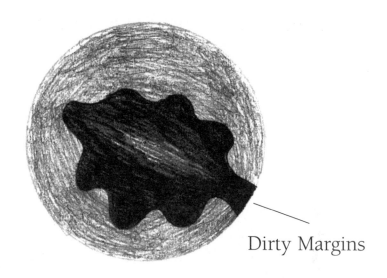

Dirty Margins

Breast Tissue That Is Removed During A Lumpectomy

Types of Surgery

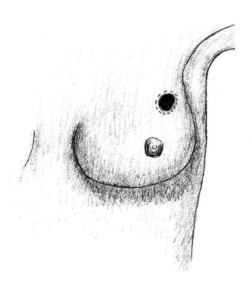

Lumpectomy

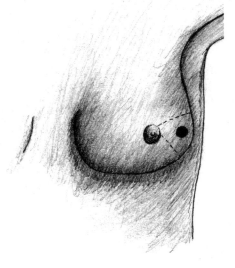

Partial Mastectomy

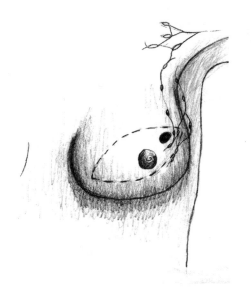

Modified Radical
Mastectomy

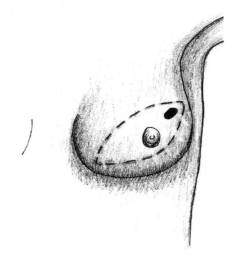

Total Mastectomy

Ductual Carcinoma Situ

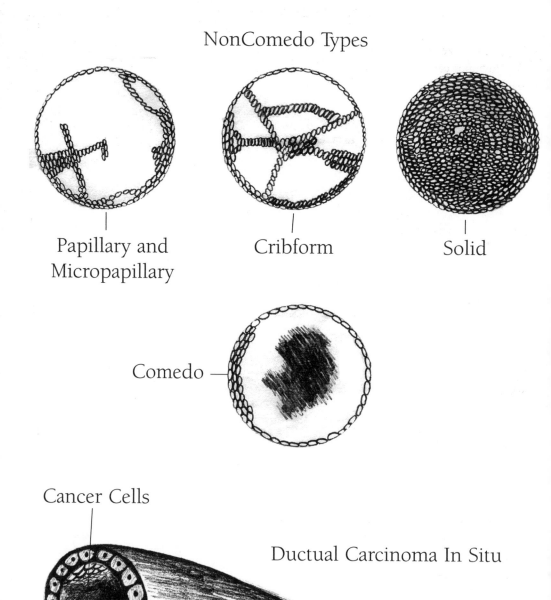

NonComedo Types

Papillary and
Micropapillary

Cribform

Solid

Comedo

Cancer Cells

Ductual Carcinoma In Situ

Wall of Duct

Breast Cancer Staging (From Life Extension):

Tumor Size*:*
TX:-Tumor size cannot be assessed.
T0:-No tumor can be found
Tis:-Only carcinoma in situ
T1:-Tumor is 2 cm or smaller
  Subcategories for T1:
  T1mic:-Very small tumor (0.1 cm or smaller)
  T1a:-Tumor is larger than 0.1 cm, but no larger than 0.5 cm
  T1b:-Tumor is larger than 0.5 cm, but no larger than 1 cm
  T1c:-Tumor is larger than 1 cm, but no larger than 2 cm
T2:-Tumor is larger than 2cm, but no larger than 5 cm
T3:-Tumor is larger than 5 cm
T4:-Tumor is any size, but has expanded past the breast tissue to the chest wall or skin
  Subcategories of T4:
  T4a:-Tumor has expanded to chest wall
  T4b:-Tumor has expanded to skin
  T4c:-Tumor has expanded to both chest wall and skin
  T4d:-Presence of inflammatory carcinoma

Lymph Node Status:
NX:- Nodes cannot be evaluated. This can happen if, for example, they have been removed previously.
N0:-Axillary nodes do not have cancer.
N1:-Axillary nodes have cancer, but can be moved
N2:-Axillary nodes have cancer and are fixed to each other or the chest wall (cannot be moved)
N3:-Internal mammary nodes have cancer
*Though classified as "early stage," prognosis can be poor for stage 2 cancers, particularly those with multiple lymph node involvement.

Distant Metastases:
MX:-Distant metastases cannot be assessed
M0:-No distant metastases
M1:-Distant metastases
  In situ cancer
Stage 0: TisN0M0
  Early Stage Invasive Cancer
Stage 1: -T1N0M0
Stage 2a: -*T0N1M0
         T1NIM0

T2N0M0

Stage 2 b*:-T2N1M0

T3N0M0

Advanced Stage Invasive Cancer

Stage 3a:-T0N2M0

TIN2M0

T2N2M0

T3N1M0

T3N2M0

3b:-T4,any N, MO

Any T, N3, M0

Metastatic Breast Cancer

Stage 4:-Any T, any N, M1

High Risk Family History:

-Keep breasts or lose breasts to surgery

-Mammograms don't work well for women with dense breasts or even younger women with dense breasts. It would help if these individuals could have any of the following tests: ultrasound, MRI, AMAS test (you pay for), or tomography (if available).

-Treatment options: radiation, chemo, or hormone blocking therapy

Genetic Breast Cancer: (BRCA1, BRCA2, BRCA3, Noey 3, and Other Rare Forms)

-Breasts being removed reduces ones risk by 90%. A woman can have emotional and cosmetic scars from this drastic procedure.

-Ovaries being removed reduces risk by 50%. The individual can't have children and but it reduces ovarian cancer by 90%.

-Treatment options: radiation, chemo, or hormone blocking therapy (For example: Tamoxifen reduces BC risk by 50% for BC women who are positive. There are side effects as hot flashes, blood clots, and the risk of endometrial cancer.)

Choices For Women With Breast Cancer:

Lumpectomy and Radiation:

-Improved psychological feelings about oneself due to less emotional scars.

-Slightly increased risk of local reoccurrence compared to a mastectomy.

-Risk of having a second surgery.

-Radiation has some temporary side effects and long term skin changes.

-Scar tissue in the effort to get clear margins from several surgeries can effect the process of re-diagnosing a patient for breast cancer.

-Additional treatment options: chemo, hormone blocking therapies, and complementary therapies

Mastectomy:

-Don't need radiation after losing a breast.

-Don't need a 2nd surgery, often times due to reduced risk of reccurence.

-There are psychological and emotional scars, sexual image issues in a relationship, and the woman feels lopsided.

-There can be a phantom breast feeling from the lost breast.

-Treatment options: chemo, hormone blocking therapies, and complementary therapies.

Bilateral Mastectomy:

-Double mastectomy with more emotional, psychological scars as well as sexual image issues.

-Phantom breast feeling from loosing two breasts.

-Probably don't need radiation.

-Treatment options: chemo, hormone blocking therapies, and complementary therapies.

Lymph Gland Tumors:

-Depending on the size of the tumor the treatment options include: surgery, radiation, chemo, and hormone blocking drugs. Nodes are positive and negative. (Tumors that are estrogen positive are treated with chemo and hormone blocking drugs depending on the risk factor and size of the tumor. Tumors that are estrogen negative are harder to treat and are often times treated with chemo.)

-There is a chance of getting lymphedema in the arm.

Advantages of Breast Reconstruction:

-You can wear bras, sports bras, swimsuits, low cut dresses, and T-shirts with comfort and ease.

-Reconstruction makes you feel like a women.

-You are not reminded of what happened to you as you look into the mirror each day.

-Reconstruction may make you feel better when you have sex as you may feel like a whole person.

Disadvantages of Breast Reconstruction:

-Reconstruction is expensive for your insurance company but is covered most often.

-There is a increased chance of infection or complications after surgery due to the surgical procedures.

-You are in the hospital longer and have more pain for a longer period of time.

When Should You Have Breast Reconstruction?

Breast reconstruction can be done at the same time as the surgical removal of your breast(s). This means only one surgery and one time in the hospital. It's cheaper, but you have more pain at one time for a longer period of time. Due to the complexity of the surgery and not having enough time to heal, you may have more complications as infections before you go on to chemo therapy. You leave the hospital feeling better about your body. You can have reconstruction sometime later when everything has healed and go through surgery again.

July 14, 2004

Dear Peggy,

Last night when we talked on the phone I could hear your concern when you asked me, "Why Me?" The only answer I can give you is my personal belief. I believe that in our journey of life we will have troubles and problems. But, what is most important is how we deal with what we're given. We must learn from these problems and meet the challenges we receive in the best way we can.

In my lung power classes, I've learned how important it is to manage the stresses in our lives. Negative feelings decrease our immunity and resistance to disease while positive feelings and emotions increase our resistance. I don't believe that stress causes cancer, but there have been studies showing that a lot of stress can cause a spreading of the cancer cells once they are there. My notes regarding that meeting included **three "C's" to help control stress:**

1.Look at changes in your life as a **challenge**. Decide what you can and should do to meet this challenge.

2.**Commitments**-Always do you the best you can for yourself, family and others.

3.Take **control** of your life by choosing positive emotions, avoid letting depression be part of your daily life.

No matter what else, each day brings something good with it, be optimistic. You have been so very strong in your battle against breast cancer. Don't let the "whys" trouble you. Just concentrate on how you will beat this disease.

Love always,

Aunt Karen

1. If you are a large breasted woman, you can save your breast.
2. You wouldn't have a reconstructed breast not matching your real breast.
3. It would be hard to have one breast and feel off balanced.
4. Psychologically and emotionally, you will feel better about yourself from a holistic stand point.
5. You can wear sports bras, bras, and no prosthesis.
6. Your breast won't float away in the swimming pool.
7. The recovery time will be shorter as will the hospital stay.

Reasons Against A Lumpectomy And Radiation

1. The grade, stage, and type of cancer would make it a poor choice.
2. There may be a high reccurence risk.
3. Radiation effects your skin color, the feel of your skin, and the texture of your skin permanently.
4. Radiation takes 5-6 weeks of treatments.
5. Your breast shrinks from radiation as well as the scar can become indented.
6. You may have a more difficult time feeling for lumps and bumps on the breast due to the skin texture.
7. If breast cancer comes back, you may need to have a second lumpectomy or a mastectomy.
8. There's been previous radiation to the chest wall, so this no longer is an option.
9. You have a large dense breast, and it wouldn't be of benefit to you.
10. The tumor is too large.
11. The location of the tumor could mean that it is not a good choice. For example, it maybe be too close to the heart to have radiation in that area.
12. You have multiple areas of microcalcifications.
13. There may be more than one tumor.
14. You're pregnant and you can't have radiation.
15. Severe medical issue may warrant not doing radiation. Examples may can include: lupus, chronic lung disease, sclerodema.

"Life will never be the same."   -Peggy Anderson

"Stand still, and consider the wondrous work of God."   -Job 37:14

"We are as much as we see."   -Thoreau's Journal

"Say it, see it, feel it!"   -Unknown Author

"What you are is God's gift to you, what you make of yourself is your gift to God."
                                                                 -Abbey Press

"Only those are fit to live who do not fear to die; and none is fit to die who has shrunk from the joy of life and the duty of life. Both life and death are parts of the same Great Adventure."   -Theodore Roosevelt

7/15/04

Dear Auntie,

I had my second surgery yesterday, and it was a lot easier than the first. After being given a local anesthesia, I walked out alert from Miller Dwan. My doctor tried to get clear margins today. Today the pain has lessened but I am taking Propoxphen. I did go over to my neighbor's house, the Strands, to get some Ibuprofen to take in between the pain pills. First I called Walgreens pharmacy and the surgical nurse at the hospital to see if I could alternate pain pills every two hours.

My surgeon, Dr. Park Skinner, called with the results. The medical and inferior margins have no tumors. There is still residual DCIS in the lateral margin. My doctor wanted to know if I wanted a simple mastectomy versus going in for another surgery on the lateral margin. I told her, " I want to try again." A surgeon can only try three times to get clear margins. After that it would be more complicated than they thought. Back to the knife!

Bad hot flashes makes sleeping hard. The Efflexor does little for me except to keep me from crying during the day. In other words, it doesn't work for hot flashes. I've gone on and off it before and after surgery. I found out that one should go off of it gradually. Oops!

I am anxious for this enemy, specifically cancer, to stop playing this game in my body. I want this battle of war with my life to end quickly. This human drama is not one in which I want to play.

Cancer patients have lots of doctor appointments and I have many. On the 19th I have an appointment with Dr. James Krook, who will be my oncologist. On the 20th I see a plastic surgeon named Dr. Dean Weber, in case all the cancer isn't gone. Then on the 26th I have surgery again on my left breast at Miller Dwan. I'll let you know what happens.

Our house is in a state of crisis and renovation. Amongst the dust and clutter Lisa, Jim, and I are still unpacking boxes and cleaning. Eric Lassila, his dad, Jerry and Jim helped with this chaotic situation to move boxes back into the of the house. Jim is starting to have back and leg problems from all the moving. One Ethan and Alan piece of furniture bled while in the outdoor storage unit due to the heat. It seems as though moisture got into the unit as there were no vents. It may be a year before every thing is in it's rightful place considering what is still left in the attic.

Life keeps unfolding with new trials. I'm tired of battling dragons and unknown feats. I'm trying to live with the BC word. How are Nancy and Steve doing going every direction with all of Brooke and Zach's activities?

Love ya,

Peggy

"Make Me Aware of People

Lord make me aware of the wonder of people. All kinds of people, old or young, important or humble, neighbor or child or foreigner or stranger on the street.

You have made us all so marvelously varied. Outwardly so different in face and form and circumstances, yet basically so much alike.

God, make me more vitally cognizant of these other worlds spinning behind all these faces. Such complex fascinating worlds, filled with memories, worries, anxieties, philosophies, and ambitions, experiences.

Remind me to listen, really listen, when people open their mouths, like small doors to that world, and try to share what's inside.

Remind me to look, really look into the hopeful windows of their eyes. I can never really enter, no, but how much I can learn from these brief glimpses. How much my own world can be expanded. (And how much I can give just by listening.)

Help me not to go coasting off on the barge of my own conceits, or wait in half-death exasperation for my turn. Help me to realize the marvel of being invited even to the doorstep of another person's world.

Lord, make me always aware of the wonder of people."

-Unknown Author

7/29/04

Dear Auntie,

I wanted to tell you the latest on what's been happening in my life. I met with my oncologist, Dr. James Krook. He is a very warm, vivacious and cordial man. Whoever said cancer is good for the soul is right. He sat on the edge of the examination table going into breast cancer with great detail. Next, he gave Jim and I the sheets of each descriptive diagram. Dr. Krook is actually someone from our past. His son, Paul, was friends with Chris at Holy Rosary. Paul and Chris went between our two houses with the wrong tennis shoes as their shoes looked alike. Dr. Krook made me laugh and cry because he is a people oriented person who finds humor in all kinds of things. He's danced with death on more than one occasion having cancer himself, and his wife had breast cancer many years ago. I felt comfortable talking to him as he's been there and come back. There is some good in all of this.

I also asked Dr. Krook about going on my trip with Kay, my sister-in-law, to South America and the Caribbean. I wanted to know if radiation and chemo could be worked around this trip, as I assured him that I had a nurse and a deacon (a spiritual advisor) going with me. Did I tell him what shape she was in? No! Did I tell him I might end up caring for her? No. She just got over pneumonia. Dr. Krook assured me we would work it out.

Dr. Krook, Jim and I discussed my chances of beating this disease and how it can improved by various treatments as surgery, radiation, chemo and hormonal therapy. We discussed my 1.5 primary breast tumor and 2 cm. auxiliary node plus extensions, HER-2/neu 2 plus positive test, the FISH test, the ER/PR positive test. I left very optimistic.

You know, I don't want to do chemo if I don't have to. For me it would be chemically alternating my body. If I have to, I will, but I don't want to. If I have a choice, I'd rather do radiation and hormone drugs. The reason being that IV needles scare me. I read on the internet about a worse case scenario where a woman got cardiomyopathy. She was fighting for her life with cancer. Well enough of Chemo 101.

One does wonder how doctors can deal with all these sad patients trying to cheer them up. Doctors have a big load to carry and hopefully they don't take on the sadness of their patients. I was determined to not be that kind of patient. My nickname is not Peggy but "Positive." I can handle this life ever changing experience.

While we were there a clinical research nurse came in to discuss clinical trials I would be qualify for. These are "free drug" and treatment trials for women. Two trials were given to me to consider, one involving drugs, and the other radiation. I will discuss these with my family doctor and the radiation oncologist at some point in time.

On the 20,[th] I saw Dr. Dean Weber from Northland Plastic and Reconstructive Surgery. I had scheduled this appointment awhile ago and wanted to follow through, in case I needed a mastectomy. The third surgery will determine if the cancer margins still aren't clear. Also, I'm doing it in case the gene test or other tests come back not looking so good at some point in time. Dr. Weber was very kind, polite and to the point as he examined me explaining the different types of breast cancer reconstructive surgery. If I end up having a breast removed I want a "tram flap." The reason being, I want my breast to look like my other breast. I have large breasts and it wouldn't look the same with a plastic breast. I was thinking about a free tummy tuck, so I can take belly dancing lessons like some Central counselors I know. I'm tired of the battle of the bulge. They remove stomach fat from this area and make a breast out of it. I was worried since I had previous cancer surgery in the pelvic area and I wouldn't qualify for this procedure. If I have a mastectomy, I want to have reconstruction at the same time. I wanted to check on the feasibility of this. Dr. Weber, a no-nonsense kind of doctor, assured me that I could have this done and he would be in contact with Dr. Park Skinner's office should it be a necessary procedure. Scheduling would be an issue as he is a very busy doctor. It would involve many hours of surgery for me as well as extensive hospitalization. Thank goodness this is covered under woman's insurance now days.

After seeing Dr. Weber, I went for another appointment to see Dr Nisswandt about my hot flashes, blood pressure, Efflexor, and over all health. I can talk to her about anything and all went well as usual.

On July 26th I had my third surgery. Oh, a nurse tried to take my blood pressure in the wrong arm as I wasn't paying attention. I need to cognizant of this and wear my medical bracelet from the American Cancer Society that states, " No IV's, blood pressure, blood tests, or injections in this arm." I'm at risk for lymphedema in this arm from having all these nodes removed. I was sent home with a prescription for Darvocet N for pain.

Then on the 28th Lisa and I went to see Diane Bierke-Nelson, a level headed Duluth Clinic genetic counselor, to have the consent forms signed for molecular DNA genetic testing (BRCA1 and BRCA 2). I had my blood drawn at this time to be sent to Myriad Medical Lab. I also had seen Diane Bierke-Nelson on the 19th and we discussed other first degree relatives who have had breast cancer. Jim went with me at this time to find out about genetic testing. Modern DNA testing! I didn't tell you what I found on the internet. It was an article that stated BRCA3 and Noey 2 are the two tests to be used if you have defective genes on your father's side of the family. Later I will ask Diane about this.

I saw Dr. Park Skinner on the 29th. Jim didn't go with as he was working. He likes to go to all of my appointments to be informed and he tells me, "In case you forget something. Four ears are better than two." Dr. Park Skinner is a great surgeon. I would go back to her in heart beat. I told her, " I feel you are my Santa Claus and you have given me a gift." She replied, " No one has told me that before." She gave me quite the gift! Dr. Skinner told me that it's not easy telling cancer patients life and death decisions, and I assured her I have had a blessed life. She told me cancer patients need to go on with their lives and not worry so much about a reoccurrence. I can go back to her if I have any concerns.

My final diagnosis showed that the surgical left lateral margin was free of tumor involvement and there was no invasive carcinoma was identified on the margins. I do have some residual cells elsewhere in the breast so I'd need radiation or chemo or both.

I think about what you said, "Peggy, this is your year of doctoring." It sure has been!

Love,

Peggy

After Surgery--What's Next? Chemo, Radiation, Hormone Therapy, Reconstruction

Cancer Facts, Terms, Knowledge, Concepts

Medical Symptoms:

Estrogen Positive Tumors-Don't eat phytoestrogens or weak estrogens, if you are estrogen positive. Ask your doctor. Cohosh and Remefemin are plant estrogens as well as soy foods, flax seeds, soy beans, and several natural estrogen supplements.

Fatigue-Signs of fatigue are dizziness, light headiness, shortness of breath, chest pains, and difficulty staying warm.

Hormone Side Effects-Hot flashes, insomnia, mood changes, and vaginal dryness are a few. (For vaginal dryness use K-Y jelly, Replens, Astroglide, or Gyne-Moistrin after talking to your gynecologist.)

Hot Flashes-Low levels of estrogen produce hot flashes, vaginal and urinary tract changes, emotional changes and osteoporosis (bone loss). Hot flashes can be treated with Primrose Oil (herbal), vitamin E or B6, plant estrogens, Propranolol (Beta Blockers), Clonidine (High Blood Pressure medicine), Cimetidine (H2 Blocker). Wear loose clothes. Talk to your doctor before taking any vitamin and herbal medicines.

Insomnia-If you can't sleep you need to address your fears by relaxing, focusing, taking life in stride, practicing deep breathing techniques and have visualizing periods of relaxation.

Mouth Sores and Care-There are several things to do if you have chemo. You should brush your teeth with a soft brush, don't visit the dentist during treatments, suck on ice or hard sugarless candy, don't eat hot, spicy and acidic foods, just eat bland foods without baking soda and yeast in it, and don't drink carbonated drinks.

Neuropathy-This is nerve damage and can occur in 1-2% of the cases. It can be caused from cancer treatments as chemo and radiation. Possible drugs that can cause neuropathy are platinum compounds, taxanes, vinca alkaloids, thalidomide, cytosine arabinoside, minonidazole, and infereron.

Infections-Preventing infections can be accomplished by washing your hands often, wearing gloves, staying away from people who are sick or coughing, don't kiss anyone, don't shake hands with people, and avoid large groups of people including sick children.

Diagnostic Procedures/Treatments:

Aromatase/Exemestane Inhibitors (ie Armidex)-This drug reduces estrogen levels in post menopausal women who are estrogen positive by blocking or shutting off the estrogen. It prevents 70-80% of all tumors in women after menopause and prevents cancer from spreading. Women need to take calcium with D when on this prescription. With Armidex you have less endometrial cancers, strokes, blood clots, vaginal bleeding, hot flashes, and discharge. You have more fractures in hip, wrist, the spine as well as other musculoskeletal disorders.

Celebrix Trials-Trial program involving Celebrix that allows you to receive free medication.

Chemo Care-This can be done by eating lightly, eating bland food, crackers, dry cereal, taking anti nausea pills, sitting up and not lying down right after eating. You should wear loose clothes when going to chemo, relax, think of pleasurable activities and take legal drugs at home.

Chemo Side Effects- Depending on the type and strength of the chemo the following may be side effects: anemia, bleeding problems, bone marrow problems, fatigue, hair loss, inability to fight infections, mouth sores, nausea, vomiting. Most of these go away and can be treated. Severe side effects of chemo are spine, thigh, and hip bone loss.

Chemo and Radiation-These two treatments can reduce the size of the tumor before surgery as they get rid of the bad cells. Radiation is in a certain area. Chemo goes all over the whole body and can't discriminate from good and bad cells.

Cocktails-Chemo cocktails kill rogue fast moving cancer cells. They can't tell the bad from the good cells.

Laparoscope-This is the removing of the ovaries through incisions. It drops cancer risk by 50%. You can still get cancer in this same place. Low dose radiation in this area and Zoladex can turn off the hormones.

Ovarian Ablation-This is the procedure where they remove both ovaries to block hormones.

Ovarian Suppression-The patient is given hormone blocker medicine to shut down the ovaries.

Ovary and Breast Removal-This has been found to reduce breast cancer by 50%.

Reconstruction of The Breast- Do's and Don'ts:

Do's- You would do reconstructive surgery because it helps you to feel better about yourself by improving your self esteem and image, gives you a permanent breast contour, provides evenness and symmetry to your breasts under your clothing, helps you to forget that you had the disease and you don't need a prosthesis.

Don't-Breast reconstruction doesn't make you look exactly like before, you don't have the same sensations as a normal breast, and it may require extra surgery to add the nipple, and the silicone breast can break open.

Reconstruction of the Breast- Pros' and Con's:

1.Implant-An implant of saline solution takes 3 hours, you're in the hospital 2 days, you usually have two drains, you have an expander that can be painful, there is scarring, it takes two weeks or more to recover, you may need a second surgery, you can't raise your arm high for a week, can't lift anything for two weeks, your chest is tight, and you have limitations for many months. There are risks with an implant as infection, it can leak, you can get lymphedema, it can turn hard, you can get capsular contracture. This procedure lasts 10-15 years and may require extra surgery. If you have radiation it can cause the skin to tighten as chemo will hinder your body to fight infection.

2.TRAM Flap-This is the most naturally shaped breast. This procedure takes 6-9 hours of surgery, you're in the hospital for a week, you have at least three drains, severe pain the abdomen requiring pain medication, recovery is six weeks to walk, tightness in stomach area, can't raise arm high for a week, can't lift and drive for 2 weeks, can't sit up or get out of bed for one week. There are risks with this surgery as the transplanted tissue can die or a seroma, fluid pocket can form by the drain. There can be a numb breast and you have no sexual stimulation. You will have weak stomach muscles as a result.

3.LATS Flap-This procedure takes 4 hours and you are in the hospital for at least 3 days. There is scaring. Recovery is 3-4 weeks, you can't raise your arm high, lift anything for two weeks, can't drive, and your chest feels tight for months. You may suffer from infection, have capsular contracture, your breast can become hard, the implant can leak, you can get lymphedema, a seroma may develop by the drain. There's no feelings in this breast. This implant lasts 10-15 years and may require additional surgery.

Risk Assessments-These are models to determine your treatment as the Gail Model and Claus Model.

Star Program- A trial program where you might be taking Tamoxifen (Nolvadex) and Raloxifene.

Systemic Treatment-Chemotherapy is a type of treatment that will go through your whole system.

Treating Breast Cancer-Do what your doctor recommends. This may include surgery, chemo, radiation, or hormone blocking therapy. Dietary modifications, detoxifications, improved diet, nutritional supplements, and vaccine therapy are other options.

Vascular Access Device (VAD)-Chemo is delivered through an implanted port in the chest wall, after being attached with a catheter that feeds to a large vein that goes back to the blood and the heart.

Medical Findings/Terminology:

Adjuvant Therapy-This is when they treat cancer that has escaped to other body parts and it is not detectable.

Antiemetic Drugs-Medicines to prevent nausea.

Autologous Tissue-The doctor reconstructs breast tissue with tissue from another part of the body.

Bone Marrow-This is where the red blood cells are produced.

Breast Enhancer- A small form that fills out the breast shape during a lumpectomy.

Breast Reconstruction-This is when a new breast is made after a mastectomy. It can be at the time of the surgery or after the surgery.

Breast Tumor-A breast tumor can grow up to 10 years before it shows its presence. This all depends on how aggressive it is.

Bilateral Mastectomy-This is when they remove both of your breasts.

Chemo Brain-The patient has trouble concentrating, is slow at processing and remembering things, loses their train of thought, can't recall, and may have cognitive decline.

Clinical Trials- Research done by using patients involved in studies to diagnose, treat, and prevent disease. The patient receives free treatments depending on the trial.

Dysesthesiae-This is pain from the part of the breast left behind.

Epogen, Procrit- Drugs to increase the production of oxygen carrying in the hemoglobin if you have chemo.

Flap-This is tissue that is attached in the original location.

Herceptin-This works to inactive Her-2/neu, a protein that makes cancer cells grow quickly. This gene accounts for 25-30% of all breast tumors. It's an IV drug that is a monoclonal antibody to target very specific proteins in the Her-2/neu. Herceptin is often used along with chemo in metastic breast cancer for women who are Her 2 neu positive. The side effects are fever, chills, shortness of breath and an increase in blood pressure. More serious side effects are nausea, weakness, pain, vomiting, headaches and rashes. In severe cases there is heart and lung damage.

Her 2/neu-These are high levels of protein found in 20-25% of all women with aggressive cancer.

LATS Flap-A latissimus dorsi flap in which tissue is removed from the upper back or side to create a breast.

Local Therapy-This is therapy that treats the tumor with surgery.

Megakaryocytes Growth Hormone-A genetic hormone that counteracts the harmful effects of chemo.

Metronomic Dosing-This is a lower dose approach to chemo.

Microvascular Surgery-The tissue is transplanted and is connected to the blood vessels.

Non-adjuvant Chemo-This is chemo that shrinks tumors like T 2 and T 3 before breast surgery.

Ovary and Breast Removal-A procedure found to reduce breast cancer by 50%.

Post-surgical bra- A breast form that sticks to you. It's similar to a self supporting bra.

Quadratectomy-This is removal of a portion of the full breast.

Saline-A salt water solution.

Segmental Mastectomy-This is a portion of the breast removed.

SERM'S (Selective Estrogen Receptor Modulators)-These mimic estrogen and bind the estrogen to receptors on cells.

Silicone- An implant bag made into a breast. Sometimes synthetic materials are used.

Systemic Therapy-This is when you choose to use chemicals (chemo) or hormone therapy to treat the cancer in your bloodstream.

TRAM Flap-A transverse rectus abdominus musculocutaneous flap. The surgeon removes tissue from the patients lower abdomen to make a surgically correct breast.

Tumor-Tumors can be benign (non-cancerous) or malignant (cancerous).

Tumor Growth-This is when the blood supply is forced to move away from healthy tissue, so that it can help the tumor to grow and feed.

Unregulated Tumor Angiogenesis- The cancer grows throughout the body.

Expander-This is a temporary implant to stretch the breast tissue to accommodate a full-size implant.

Xeloda-This is an oral chemo for metastic breast cancer.

Zofan ODT-This is an anti nausea medicine.

Medical Reports/Doctors:

Plastic Surgeon-This is a doctor that does reconstructive surgery on the breast.

Reconstruction

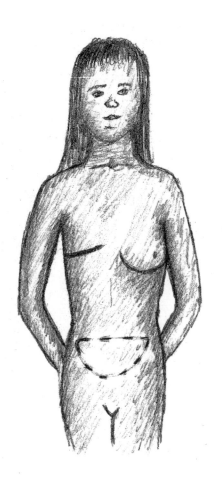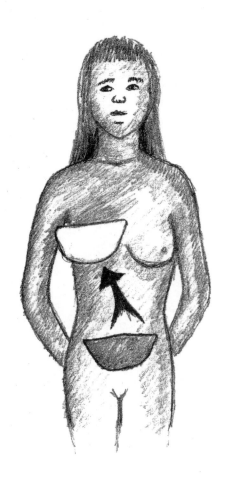

Tram Flap

Reconstruction

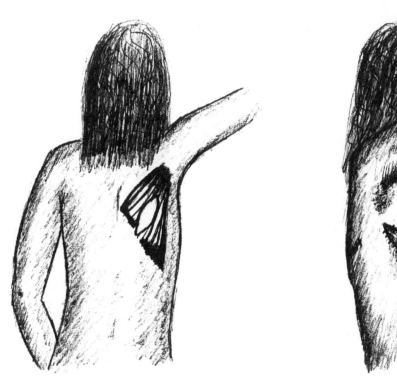

Latissimus Flap Surgery

Implant on Reconstructed Breast

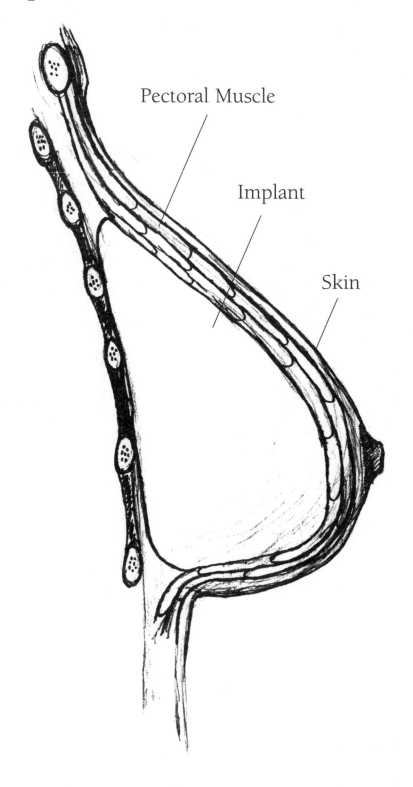

Pectoral Muscle

Implant

Skin

August 3, 2004

Dear Peggy,

We'll have to mark our calendars that on July 26th was a special day. Peggy's breast margins are finally clear of cancer cells! How thankful we all are for the skills of your surgeon.

Last week Jim and I met Jean McFarlin for brunch at the Cracker Barrel. Jean had a mastectomy in 1972. Her doctor removed seven lymph nodes without finding additional cancer and no recommendation was made for further treatments. There's been no reoccurrence in the past twenty-three years. Another example how this disease can be conquered.

Jean and I met in kindergarten at Washburn School in Duluth. This past Valentine's Day her husband Joe died from complications of melanoma cancer. Unfortunately, not all battles with cancer are won. Medical science has come far in the study and treatment of cancer but much still needs to be accomplished. We need to support further cancer research to give our physicians more tools and knowledge to work with. Joe was a KDAL announcer in Duluth until they moved to Minneapolis where he worked for WCCO until he retired.

I so well remember my last visit with Joe in the fall of 2003. Marylu Young, my dear friend forever from kindergarten days, came down from Chub Lake to spend a few days with me after my trip to the hospital for colitis and pneumonia. Remember that's when I blew a hole in my colon.

Jean and Joe met Marylu, my Jim and I at the Edinburgh Clubhouse for lunch. We spent hours talking. It was such a beautiful fall day that we ended up on our deck that my son-in-law, Steve and his father had rebuilt for us this summer. I was very touched by Delane's helping. He's fighting his own battle with cancer. I brought out a few of my many photo albums of us girls in school, our dating days and marriages. We have a lot of history together going back over seventy years.

Before Jean and Joe left I opened a bottle of champagne to toast our many memories. Joe didn't want to drink because of his medications but I quietly told him that, " The best is yet to come." He asked me if I really believed that and I assured him I did by saying, "One way or another." I wasn't able to visit him those last few months as I was again in bed with another case of pneumonia.

Today was a great day. Marylu and Tom drove down to take us to lunch at the Edinburgh Clubhouse, a belated celebration of my 76th birthday on July 30.th Marylu and I have exchanged gifts since we were kids. Her gifts are always a reflection of her and are very thoughtful and special. When walking through my home, many rooms bring a special memory of this dear friend. These gifts have ranged from the oil painting of birches she did the first year we moved here and to the beautiful watercolor of geraniums she did for my 75th that greets me each morning. On her card was a magnet for the refrigerator, "Friends Forever." The friends we make in our life can so enrich our well being. I've been blessed with some that go back to my childhood school days. But, I have concern that today with so many women holding full time jobs as well as raising a family, and keeping up their homes that they won't have time to nourish these relationships. Women friends are always ready to share their experiences, talk with you about your problems, give suggestions, and be a strong support in your life. This letter has gotten very long but I wanted to share these stories with you.

Love always,

Auntie Karen

"The best and most beautiful things in the world cannot be seen or touched--but are felt in the heart."   -Helen Keller

"Has any man attained inner harmony by pondering the experience of others? Not since the world began! He must pass through the fire."   -Norman Douglas

"He who is plenteously provided from within, needs but little from without."
                                          -Johann Wolfgang von Goethe

"Come to me, all you who are weary and burdened, and I will give you rest."
                                          -Matthew 11:28

"Kind words can be short and easy to speak, but their echoes rare… truly endless."
                                          -Mother Teresa

8/6/04

Dear Auntie,

At this time I want to report to you how things are going. Tuesday night I went to my first Breast Cancer Support group meeting. It happened to be an open discussion, and I met some exceptionally nice people. A couple of women who had cancer 12-13 years ago were at this meeting. One women knew Kay very well. Hearing other women's stories helps me to understand the types of cancer they have had and what treatment choices they've made. Some have been through hell and back. Support group has speakers throughout the year as well as open discussion meetings at Miller Dwan, and they serve snacks. I plan on going once a month to this group.

How am I feeling? I'm feeling like I need a road map to my mind's thinking. It must be stress, as I feel like my thoughts are swimming away at the river bank. I'm getting more forgetful, maybe from not sleeping at night.

Jim is having excruciating sciatica problems. I believe it is from moving all of the furniture in and out of our house. We had our wood floors refinished by Larsen Flooring and they did an excellent job! Jim saw Dr. Lillegard, my favorite very perceptive orthopedic doctor, who I've seen many times. He's going to physical therapy and doing exercises many times a day. To say the least, he is very miserable.

I picked up the drapes as soon as they were cleaned, and it was quite the stitch to see the two of us trying to hang them up. Jim with his sciatica problem and me with my stitches in two places.

Here's a few sound bites from my puppies. Smokey Joe and Peanut Butter had their hair cuts at Amity Kennels, or should I say as Annie does, "They're going to get naked." They get real excited to go to Aunt Annie's. She's a first class dog lover and even kisses them. Who wouldn't ask for aunt like her?

On Wednesday I had a travel center appointment to find out what shots I needed for the Panama cruise with Kay. It was recommended that I bring Cepro, have a flu and pneumonia shot due to my immune system. I could get a letter to get out of malaria shot, but I may need a yellow fever shot after I recheck with the travel agency. (It depends how far we go into the rain forest.) All my hepatitis shots are up to date from being a teacher and our traveling.

I'm thinking that I can lose some weight on my trip. Maybe, I can do some real walking and come back as a lean, mean fat burning machine. I'll really have to watch what I eat, if it's anything like the Royal Caribbean Christmas cruise we went on. Jim would like me to come back as the energized bunny who is always moving and going places with him. Right now my energy level is real poor.

I wish I could eat sugar, but I know that it's not good for a cancer patient. Sugar is a problem in America. Americans drink too much pop and sugar laced products, so they are getting diseases. It's a wake up call when it happens.

In reading, I came across an article that stated women who are in your age category and who have low levels of serum total and bioavailability estradiol have bone mineral density problems of the femur, spine and in their total body. It's a good thing you are on estrogen therapy, but I wonder if you are on the right therapy, so you don't get osteoporosis down the road.

Love and kisses,

Peggy

August 10, 2004

Dear Peggy,

I was so excited to learn from your last letter that your plans to cruise to Panama in November are working out.

These past months have been so stressful for both you and Jim that you need a break. I think all this stress and worry is stirring up Jim's health problems. You need something good to look forward to. I know Jim will be lonesome, but I also know Jim wants you to be happy.

I hope you make the trip a "celebration of life," a chance to enjoy new adventures and time to reflect on the goodness of life.

You asked me about Steve's dad, Delane, and his battle with cancer. In the spring of 2000, he went in for a routine physical and after various tests he ended up having surgery for kidney cancer. His surgeon told him to get his affairs in order as there was nothing more they could do for him. Pat made an appointment for Del at Parker Hughes Clinic in the cities. They use very advanced and aggressive treatment to fight cancer. His chemo was rough--miserable erps, diarrhea, swelling of the body, and while under treatment he lost his hair. He is now busy fishing, building Zach a tree house and enjoying life. The clinic is monitoring him by CAT, MRI and PET scans. He will return to chemo if needed. Del is not a quitter. Both Pat and Del are very grateful to Parker Hughes for giving him this second chance of life. This shows the importance of never losing hope and why a second opinion is often necessary.

Another example of the importance of second opinions happened while Delane was still undergoing treatments. Pat's sister, Penny, was also diagnosed with cancer and was scheduled for throat surgery to remove her voice box. Penny lives in Montevideo, and Pat convinced her to come to the cities to get a second opinion at Parker Hughes before losing her voice. She stayed with Pat and Del while undergoing chemo. Pat once remarked, it was the "Larson Nursing Home," and she was glad they had two bathrooms. Today she is also being monitored by Parker Hughes, has her voice and feels wonderful.

Nancy and Steve won't be taking a summer vacation trip this year. Their busiest times are at opposite ends of the calendar. Starting in spring, Steve puts in long days supervising lane closures and detours for new highway construction, big repair jobs and special events.

Nancy is using her summer break time to get caught up at home with all the things she has to skip during her busy school year. Also, there's time to do some extra fun things with her kids. I don't think she plans on taking any extra classes in the summer until her children are older. I can remember how every summer you would take on summer school teaching. You didn't leave much time for yourself.

You and I both know how important it is that our teachers have this long break to "re-charge" for the next school year. Nancy is like you always were, Peggy, going at full speed for her students. In raising my family I remember how, by the end of the summer, they were eager for that first day back at school. But by May, the "drag" would set in. Also, at the spring conferences it would sometimes be with a crabby teacher. Students and teachers need the long summer breaks to revitalize education.

Brooke missed so many kindergarten days, or had to leave school early due to her asthma, that she's been going to a catch-up class for six weeks. She enjoyed having her Mom drive her each morning and pick her up at noon. Trips to the community pool are her favorite as she adores swimming.

Zach had a great time at hockey camp. I worried about my nine year old grandson staying at St. Cloud University. It was such a hot week, no A/C in the dorm, and the kids had a long hike to the college's ice arena. But, he's already making plans to go back next year.

Keep me posted on your treatments and remember to always keep positive.

Love always,

Aunt Karen

"Happy families are all alike, every unhappy family is unhappy in it's own way."
-Anna Karenia

"When one door of happiness closes, another opens; but often we look so long at the closed door that we do not see the one which has opened for us."   -Helen Keller

"If I were asked to give what I consider the single most useful bit of advice for all humanity it would be this: Expect trouble as an inevitable part of life and when it comes, hold your head high, look it squarely in the eye and say, "I will be bigger than you. You cannot defeat me."   -Ann Landers

"When God closes a door, He always opens a window."   -Ganz

"For he shall give his angels charge over you, and keep you in all your ways."
-Psalm 91:11

8/13/04

Dear Auntie,

Life has changed the way that I look at it today. I hope you're not getting tired

of me talking about "BC." My discussing it is probably getting as repetitive as a

Lutheran Hymnal. This has been an especially busy week for Jim. He's been going to

physical therapy, had dentist appointments and Ham Radio activities.

We met with Dr. Krook, my oncologist, on Tuesday, and he was glad that Dr. Park

Skinner got the last margin. We discussed clinical trials and treatment for breast

cancer again. Dr. Krook was optimistic and funny as usual. He estimated my long

term remission at 75-80% but then added, if I did hormone blocking medication, and

radiation it would be 85%. Chemo would only raise it to 86-87 % at the most. Dr.

Krook told me his colleagues would also advise standard chemotherapy because of the

one positive node, but I chose not to do it for so low a percentage. I was concerned

about long term effects from chemo depending on the type and the strength. He

assured me he could mix a weak chemo comination (chemo cocktail) but I didn't want

to do it. I realize the pros and cons of chemo. The good part about chemo is you

could lose your hair, if you want a bald head, your hair may return curly hair or even a

122

different color! This recalled in my memory something that Lisa once me. This was something that one of Mary Dwan's daughters said to her when her hair turned a different color. She said, "You're not my mother." He assured me I wouldn't have any strong chemo, but I still think chemo is a choice to be used down the road, if necessary. There are risks with regional cancer and not doing chemo. I decided on the radiation and taking Armidex, which is a armonstate inhibitator for metastic breast cancer. I feel good about my choice and I'm willing to take the chance of delaying chemo in the hopes of avoiding it. After talking to Dr. Krook, I realized how important wit and humor still are in this world. He is sure a source of courage and strength.

I wanted to tell you about three articles I read about having a lumpectomy versus a mastectomy. One was in the *New England Journal of Medicine* on 10/17/02. In the article, it stated there were a number of clinical trials in which women with invasive breast cancer were treated with mastectomy or lumpectomy and radiation. The outcome showed that they were equally effective in survival and reccurrence. Then another study reported in a magazine article from *Dartmouth Medical School* (92-93) showed the same results. A third magazine article stated that *Harvard Medical School* had up to 70% lumpectomy breast operations in comparison to 1.4% in Rapid City, S.D.

As I was scanning the internet today, I found an article from *Allegheny University* that had done studies on women who had DCIS with comedo or comedo necrosis. They can predict the cancer's reoccurrence from the dead cells. Since I had invasive cancer and DCIS with comedo, it seems I may have a recoccurence. I also read somewhere on a report that I had solid, crib form focal necrosis, proliferate breast disease, ductual epithelia hyperplasia, multimodal. It makes me wonder what this all means. I see why some women don't want to worry about this, and they go straight to the mastectomy instead of facing it down the road. I'm having body hot flashes. Peggy

" The Extravagance of God
More sky than man can see,
    More sea than he can sail,
        More sun than he can bear to watch,
        More stars than he can scale.
            More breath than he can breathe,
                More yield than he can sow,
                    More grace than he can comprehend,
                    More love than he can know."
                                            -R.W. Seager

8/20/04

Dear Auntie,

Here's the latest and have I been busy. I saw Dr. Mike Bussa on Monday. My teeth needed to be taken care of before I start radiation, as I read in an article that you should see the dentist before radiation and chemo. Tuesday I went to our annual luncheon with former Duluth School special education teachers and personnel at Porters Restaurant. It was fun getting together. Ellen Moore Anderson discussed her book, *As Long as The Moon Shall Rise* that will be coming out soon. On Wednesday I went to the book sale at the Duluth Public Library. Then on Thursday I went for my allergy shot, and later met with Dr. David Frye, my radiation oncologist, at Miller Dwan Hospital.

Off to Radiation 101. Dr. Frye is young, a vibrant doctor that mesmerizes you with his knowledge of information, and he wants to do his very best for you. Jim was impressed with him as well. I brought along some of my medical records, as I thought he would want to know that I had two cysts in my neck as a baby. At that time I had two deep x-ray radiation treatments. It turns out that he is the first doctor that could tell me what was wrong with my neck. I have tell-tale signs of previous radiation treatments, and he decided I should have a thyroid test.

Patients have to sign a paper that will allow pictures to be taken by way of a closed circuit television for medical purposes. Also, the additional risks from radiation were explained to me. They include fatigue, skin irritations, the feeling of a lump in the throat, difficulty or pain in swallowing, increase in cough or heartburn. The long term risks are radiation pneumonitis (inflammation of the lung), and radiation fibrosis (scarring of the lung tissue). Radiation over radiation can cause radiation fibrosis, and this is one of Dr. Frye's biggest challenges. There is potential for lymphedema in the left arm as well. Other risks may include a possible rib breaking or heart problems. But treatments completely avoid the heart with such accurate measurements now days. I need to go back next week to be measured as everything has to be extremely accurate. They take pictures, do extensive measurements once a week, besides measuring each time you have a treatment. The first time I will be there the longest.

I feel like I'm in a labyrinth trying to find the way out to the causes of my cancer, and the timer is clicking. The pathway is too confusing because I don't know if I should go to the left or to the right. I desperately want the answer to this puzzle. Time is of the essence, I need to get out, and find the cause of this disease.

There are many factors that play into cancer treatment. They include surgery, chemo, radiation, and hormone blocking therapy. Treatment is not the only factor in the equation. The whole person is very important (body, mind, and spirit). For example, we need to be our own advocates to work with doctors to find the cause of the cancer. I believe that the conditions in our body set the stage for cancer like a stage of a theater is set for a play.

Knowledge of preventive information, as well as causes can help the patient to have a longer and better prognosis. For example, is one having hormone or adrenal gland imbalance problems? Is the patient eating a healthy diet and maintaining normal body mass? How does an individual deal with life stressors and emotional hang-ups? What environmental toxins has a person been exposed to? What is a person's family health and cancer history? A patient should be asked, "What do you think is the cause of your cancer?" Maybe cancer patients need a few more tests or questionnaires. Initial causes can be psychological, emotional, physical, or nutritional. There can be several reasons that the stage was set for cancer.

I read somewhere that doctors try to remove all the cancer, but at what cost to the body? Maybe we don't have to use such radical treatments which can have side effects down the road or maybe we do. People's bodies need to be like piano pieces from practice. A bad key ruins the piece like a cancer cell caused from a mutation. Treatment should prevent errors in the performance, stop cancer reccurrences, or any major disaster within the body. It's also a way that no one can be blamed. The patient survives living happy ever after or until the next reccurence comes along from not changing the cause of the problem. (Dr. Quillin's book has had an effect on my life!)

I've thought about what could of possibly caused my cancer. Mine could be from..

- **poor diet-**(High red meat, high saturated fats, high dairy, not enough fruits, vegetables, and grains may have caused problems with my immune system to not fight this DNA mutation hit.)

-**stressors in my life-**(I admit I'm a type A driven, work alcoholic type person. There's been stressors in my life that may of worn down my immune system and released cortical: growing up in a dysfunctional family, working full time while going to college, being an over achiever, raising my own family, a job and graduate school.)

-**previous cancers-**(I've had cervical cancer and then bad cells again.)

-**previous high dose ionizing x-rays and mammograms-**(2 deep x-rays to my neck at 3 months; at least 3 chest x-rays before age 17; 11 chest x-rays before age 32; mammograms late 30's on) I had scoliosis as a child, fell from the 2nd floor to the first floor as a child, have been in two car accidents where the vehicles were totaled, one ski accident, etc.

-**a previous biopsy where bad cells could have been missed due to a blood vessel breaking**

-**or the cancer that didn't show up on the mammogram-**(I have dense breasts.)

-**inflammation in my left side of my chest wall that couldn't be diagnosed**

-**or hormonal imbalance-**My tumor is estrogen/progesterone positive. (I took

Estradiol, Premarin, and Estradiol over the years for HRT. I was on low

doses in my later years.)

-maybe from not sleeping at night- (Possibly, I could had melatonin issues for the

past six months from Ham radio equipment. I've had trouble sleeping, that's for

sure.)

-eating a lot of soy products one month before I was diagnosed-(This probably

wasn't the cause.)

-being around oil and gasoline as a child- (My Father owned Prahl Oil Company,

and we had a tank at our house so we were around fuel and oil.)

-maybe over using antibiotics in years past

-being excessively overweight which caused too much estrogen in my body

-household toxins and products-(I used scrubbing cleaners with bleach, turpentine,

rubber cement, plastic baggies, plastic wrap, washed my counters with bleach water,

chlorine and bromine (pool or hot tub), certain chemicals in beauty products, a lot of

bleached paper as a teacher, and two times cleaned our pool with bleach.)

Mutagens can increase mutations of DNA. There's carcinogens that are

environmental agents which lead to cancer. They are mutagenic and they include

chemicals, organic causes, radiation, and viruses. Organic chemicals would be like

fat and estrogen (HRT) promoting breast cancer. (If you're not estrogen dominant

you don't need to worry.) Remember there is excessive estrogen in our body fat.

Chemicals could also include cigarette smoke, saccharin, number two red dye, and

industrial chemicals such as benzene, carbon tetrachloride, vinyl chloride, and

asbestos fiber. Pesticides, herbicides, dioxin can also fall into this category as well.

Radiation can occur from various types of radiation, x-rays, nuclear bombs, power

plants, radon in homes, UV sunlight, and tanning lights. Viruses can include hepatitis

and retroviruses. Cancer can even show up in people who are immune compromised

as you, Auntie. We all get cancer. Dr. Quillin states in his tape that, "Forty-two

percent of the people can't fight cancer off. The other fifty-eight percent of the people can fight the cancer in their body!"

When I think of our bodies, I start thinking of them as vegetable gardens. With a garden, we first need good soil, but still we need to remove the rocks and weeds. Next we plant our vegetables, add plant nutrients, and shower the vegetables with water. The sun and good quality soil are antioxidants. We use tender loving care with our green thumbs, hoping and praying the plants will grow fruitfully. Our bodies have a body burden of chemical toxins in them. I read somewhere that the more fluids you drink the better it is for removing toxins in the body, but I haven't researched this out. Also in regard to our psychological health, the thoughts, words, feelings we all carry around bottled up inside of us need to be released as well. We add nutrients and water to our body, hoping it will suffice our daily needs and make us immune strong. Some of us may overindulge our bodies with junk and fast foods that leads the way to diseases. We pull the weeds diligently out of the garden, but we can't get them out of our bodies until we have surgery. We need to use more tender loving care with our bodies, our temples, when we make daily choices in food, to avoid stressors, and make quality living choices.

I am like a cat with nine lives. I had In Situ Squamous Carcinoma of the uterine cervix with dysphasia, cervictis, and metaplasia in 1971. Then years later I had bad cells in that area left over that caused hemorrhaging and ulceration problems. I was sent to the Mayo Clinic a few times. Dr. Bill Jaccott, my accomplished family doctor at the time, had a gynecologist in town use cryotherapy on this area and the problem was solved. Didn't you have cervical cancer?

Next week is a busy week for me as I have to go to Miller Dwan for measurements and will be there for awhile. Also, I must meet with Diane Bierke-Nelson to go over my genetic testing. Then on the Friday and Saturday Lisa and I are having a multi family garage sale. Call when you are available.

Love,

Peggy   Enclosed is some more cancer information.

Cancer Facts, Terms, Knowledge, Concepts

Symptoms:

Brachial Plexopathy-This is a form of peripheral neuropathy. It occurs in the brachial plexus where the nerve bundles split. Nerve damage can occur from radiation and often is the result of a lack of oxygen in this area.

Costochondritis-Inflammation and pain around the thin covering of the ribs.

Dry Mouth-This occurs from lack of salvia and can cause damage to teeth and gums.

Radiation Headaches-An infrequent symptom and there may be associated symptoms as nausea, irritability, and loss of appetite. Siberian ginseng sometimes helps this problem but ask your doctor first.

Typical Side Effects of Radiation:

-Fatigue, loss of appetite, sunburn, itchiness, redness, swelling, blistering, and decreased sensation (hyper sensation), shrinking of skin, and color discoloration can occur.

Rare Side Effects from Radiation:

-Rib fracture or susceptibility (1%), lung damage and inflammation (1%), swelling and heaviness in the arm, nerve damage (brachial plexopathy), sarcoma (rare), heart damage (not with new machines), low blood count (lymphocytes and platelets drop), leukemia (risk of dying from original disease is higher), radiation fibrosis and scarring from atrophy of tissues (You should treat these tissues gently the rest of your life.), carcinogenicity (Radiation is the cause of cancer.), hypertension in lymph areas and a stroke.

-**Radiation Fibrosis** is a thickening of the skin. It can occur after radiation in up to a year after treatments. It often occurs when radiation overlaps previous radiation treatments in an area and is irreversible.

-**Radiation Pneumonitis**-This is when there is inflammation of the lung (s) due to radiation. It occurs 2 weeks to 6 months after therapy and is reversible with a cortisone drug such as prednisone. The symptoms are cough, fever and it is confirmed by x-rays.

Diagnostic Procedures/Treatments:

Adjuvant Therapy-A treatment given after a primary treatment.

Brach therapy (Brachtherapy/Interstitial Therapy)-They plant radioactive seeds into a specific area after you have had a lumpectomy. This procedure often takes place while you are hospitalized in a private room and takes 4-5 days versus 6 weeks of radiation. After this the implants are removed.

External Beam Radiation-This is high energy radiation that is done to the breasts and nodes after surgery. It involves particle waves aimed at the breast cells coming at you from different directions as you lie on a table for radiation treatments. It doesn't hurt. Length of treatments vary, but typically you go 10-30 minutes a day, five days a week, for 5-6 weeks.

Hyerfractionated Radiation Therapy-A time when daily doses are separated into smaller doses for radiation therapy.

Internal Radiation-Radiation within the body, it can be from radiation seeds in the breast.

Lymphedema Precautions-Don't restrict your arm, avoid heat, hot sun and burns, take care of your skin in the winter and summer, avoid scratches and pet bites, don't shave under your arm, treat cuts immediately, use antibiotics, avoid tight clothing or restriction on the arm or the lymphedema area, avoid muscle strain by not lifting anything over 10-20 pounds, and wear a lymphedema bracelet with the four precautions on it.

Mammograms-Mammograms deliver ionizing radiation. The risk of cancer accumulates in the body after each exposure. Women who have genetic issues, those who come from a family that is high risk, and women who start mammograms early on are more at risk. Today mammograms are low dose.

Mammosite RTS/Balloon Brachtherapy-This is partial breast irradiation, and it's a procedure when the doctor plants a spherical balloon catheter into your breast after a lumpectomy to deliver high doses of radiation. This procedure delivers the radiation only to a specific area, so that other healthy tissue isn't damaged. A procedure like this takes five days. It is for early stage breast cancer, the lump has to be a certain size, and your lymph nodes must be negative.

Managing Side Effects from Radiation:

Radiation Nausea-Avoid greasy and salty foods, eat small frequent meals, drink ice cold drinks.

Fatigue/Malaise- Put your feet up, get plenty of rest by taking naps, have regular blood tests to test your red blood cells and lymphocytes.

Appetite-Eat healthy.

Clothing-Wear loose shirts, a T-shirts, no bra, and avoid tight clothing in the treatment area(s).

Irritated Skin-If red or uncomfortable ask the doctor for a medicated cream.

Pain, Fever, Cough, Sweating-Tell your doctor if you have these symptoms!

Other Experimental Therapies-These include partial breast radiation and intra-operative radiotherapy.

Skin Problems During Treatments:

-avoid deodorant, perfume, heat, dust, trauma, open air

-use non-stick dressings

-use corn starch under the arm, if allowed

-avoid direct sunlight to the treatment area

Radiation-Radiation is either external or internal high energy x-rays treatments. You can be either stage I, II, III, or IV and have radiation. Radiation has been used with a lumpectomy as well as mastectomy. In some cases it is used to stop the spread of metastasis.

Radiation Do and Don'ts: You shouldn't rub the treatment area, but do wash it with mild soap and lukewarm water, only do sponge baths or short showers, use moisturizers, wear loose cotton tops, don't wear bras, don't use a razor, use an electric razor when allowed, don't shave under your arm, no hot tubs, no chlorinated pools, don't use antiperspirant or deodorant, use corn starch if allowed, protect your skin from the cold, don't scratch your skin, and keep out of sun. Only do what your physician recommends.

Reducing Side Effects for Radiation and Chemo-Vitamin E reduces toxicity; Vitamin C reduces side effects and protects bone marrow, Coenzyme Q10 or CoQ10 helps to prevent cell damage from chemo as it's an antioxidant. Ask your doctor first before taking any vitamins or pills.

Medical Findings/Terminology:

Acute-Short term during treatment.

Alpha-Cradle-Device that positions you to keep you in the correct place during radiation.

Block-A template is made, so there's accurate measurements of your treatment area. It's inserted into the linear accelerator (x-ray machine).

Chronic-Long term means it may be permanent.

CT Scans-Imaging studies of a specific body part.

Desquamation-This is the crusting of skin from erythematic to dry desquamation and moist desquamation. Healing occurs from underneath the skin.

Electron Beam-Often used to boost treatments in a targeted area.

Ionizing Radiation/High Dose (Radioactive Radiation)-This kind of radiation increases your chances of getting breast cancer. Children who have radiation at an early age or as a young adult can get breast cancer later in life.

Linear Accelerator-A machine in which you lie on the table to have your breast cancer treatments.

Other Types of Radiation Treatment-Hyper fractionated radiation therapy, dimensional conformal radiation therapy, and precision therapy are other types.

Radiation (Radiotherapy) (RT), X-ray Therapy or Irradiation-Radiation is delivered by a large machine called a linear accelerator that delivers precise amounts of high-energy radiation by way of x-rays, electron beams, or cobalt-60 gamma rays. It is used to kill renegade cancer cells. This type of radiation minimizes damage to healthy tissues. Radiation has shown to improve a woman's survival rate.

Sarcoma-This is a cancer that starts in the connective tissue such as a bone, cartilage or muscle.

Scarring of Lungs-This can occur if you have chronic pneumonitis.

Simulation-A simulation is when you can receive your treatment from a port or field on the table.

Telangiectasis-These are small, red areas that can appear in 10-12 months after radiation from dilated blood vessels. Your skin may change in color or fade, and there could be changes in the size, and shape to your skin.

Tumor Bed (Lumpectomy Cavity)-This is the tissue surrounding the spot where the tumor was.

Medical Reports/Radiation Health Care Professionals:

Other People Involved-These could be the social worker, dietician, physical therapist, physicians assistant, chaplain or spiritual director.

Radiation Dosimetrists-These individuals calculate the number and length of treatments. They work under the direction of a doctor and radiation physicist to calculate the amount of radiation delivered.

Radiation Nurse-The nurse is certified to take care of you, is an individual who understands your treatments, and has knowledge of the side effects.

Radiation Oncologist-A doctor who specializes in radiation cancer treatments. He will determine what therapy you will have, monitors you, and adjusts your progress.

Radiation Physicist-This is the person who works with the radiation oncologist to look at your measurements to make sure they are very accurate. He makes sure the equipment works and corrects the radiation dosage and delivery.

Radiation Therapists-These are the people who set up treatments each day and run the x-ray machines.

Radiologist-This is the person who reads and interprets the x-rays.

Computer Generated Radiation Dose Treatment In The Breast

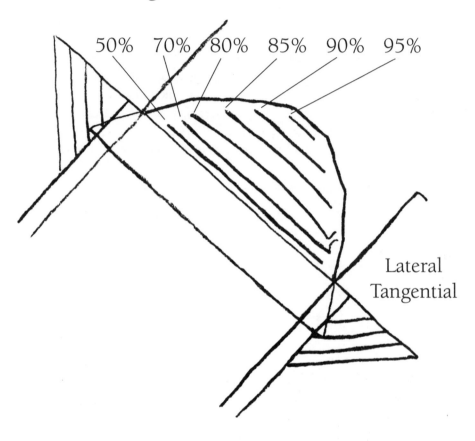

Medial Tangential

50% 70% 80% 85% 90% 95%

Lateral
Tangential

Linear Accelerator

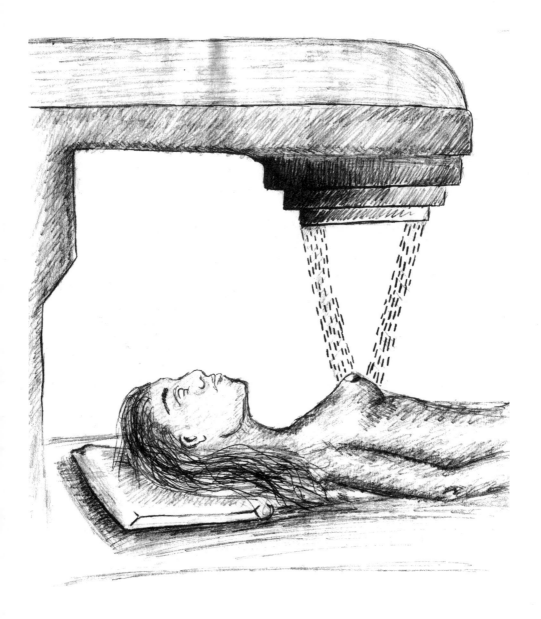

Minor Side Effects:
Skin irritation
Redness, like a sunburn

Short Term or Long Term:
Cracking of skin
Skin infection
Breast swelling
Nausea
Irritability
Soreness
Poor appetite
Fatigue, from healing and going five days a week
Stress of going to treatments and having breast cancer
Dry mouth
Coughing
Swallowing, if lymph nodes are being treated
Low blood count
Radiation Pneumonitis (rare)
Rib breaking

Very Long Term/Permanent/Very Rare:
Lymphedema
Brachial Plexopathy
Radiation Fibrosis-irreversible
Lung damage
Sarcoma
Heart Damage, but not with new machines
Tissue scarring
Hypertension
Leukemia
Cancer

Radiation Therapy

The purpose of radiation is to damage the cancer cells which grow in a low oxygen environment. Reversing hypoxia or providing more oxygen to cancer to help radiation work is very important. Radiation allows more free radicals to effect the cancerous tumor(s).

"You gain strength, courage, and confidence by each experience in which you really stop to look fear in the face. You are able to say to yourself, "I have lived through this horror. I can take the next thing that comes along."   -Eleanor Roosevelt

"Diseases can be our spiritual flat tires-discrepancies in our lives that seem to be disasters at the time, but end by redirecting our lives in a meaningful way."
                                                        -Bernie S. Siegel, M.D.

"The Lord is my light and my salvation-whom shall I fear? The Lord is the stronghold of my life-of whom shall I be afraid."   -Psalm 27:1

"It is by grace you have been saved."   -Ephesians 2:5

"I can live two months on one good compliment."   -Mark Twain

"Be angry, but do not sin; do not let the sun go down on your anger." -Ephesians 4:26

9/7/04

Dear Auntie,

    Well, I'm down the mountain and on the road again. Today I saw Dr. Nisswandt, my down to earth, natural family doctor. Try to picture my doctor with long hair, that usually is back, and she wears long skirts. Anyhow, she answered my numerous questions that I spit out one right after another. Wasn't it Albert Schweitzer that once said, "Each patient comes with a doctor inside of him?" I'm not trying to play doctor, I'm just trying to find the answers.

    Today I had my radiation simulation appointment. A whole new paradigm was set for me on August 25th. Before I could begin treatments they had to map out by pinpointing the exact location of my breast and lymph cancer. First I had to lay on the CT simulator (computerized tomography scanner) table with a breast board. Next they did axial images and measurements to set up the treatment areas. They develop a special, customized designed pillow block to hold you in place after all the air has been sucked out of it. It forms a mold for your head and arm as you are immobilized. Radiation reuses these expensive molds by letting air back out and in. Dr. Frye measured me as the therapist put permanent tattoos on me. (Oh, mine are not the same color as Dr. Krook's.) After all this measuring, they send this information to the physicist and dosimetrist to examine the results, so they can plan out the measurements, dose of radiation and how long the beam will be. It seemed like this procedure took about an hour, and it was quite amazing, not scary.

My radiation treatments began a few days later. A radiation therapist told me to take my shirt off and lay on the table. She covered the area not to be treated with a cloth as they precisely measure each time. Another technician asked, "Do you want to listen to music during treatment?" My answer was, "Sure." They played *The Righteous Brothers.*

The two technicians leave the room, turn on the linear accelerator, deliver the radiation as they view you on a television monitor. It takes 1-30 minutes for all of the radiation steps. The nurses and technicians are always friendly, talkative, and overall jubilant with all their patients.

Dr. Frye told me when I have super boost treatments at the end, it will involve at least seven sessions. This will be on the tumor areas to prevent a chance of reccurrence. I read some studies on the internet that stated women who have radiation after a lumpectomy have a higher survival rate. Also, I read that women 70 and older often don't do radiation. Remember I had deep x-ray radiation at 3 months and I'm still alive 56 years later!

At times when I go to radiation, I see patients that remind me of the book, *Night,* that I use to read with my English classes. I recall the look and the loss of spirit. The patients are cheered up by the technicians greeting them and bringing them into treatment rooms.

Today I turned in my family medical sheets to Miller Dwan. The form requested information about my immediate family, my Mother's side, my Father's side and who had various cancers and their ages. The cancers they wanted to know about were breast, ovarian, prostrate, pancreatic, male breast cancer, and any other cancers within the family structure. I guess we should all be keeping this information in our medical files.

Breast Cancer Support group at Miller Dwan is tonight, and I need to bring a blanket as we will be doing Yoga mediation. I think it should be fun. It's the time of the month that I realize I am not the only vulnerable person on this earth. We all have to be very resilient to the differences of others. We need to look where we have been, and where we are going. Some individuals have real vision and clarity on what has happened to them. Some are stuck in the muck and can't get out. Others have returned to their purpose in life showing the strength to rebuild their lives. I know, I just want a return to the rest of my life without cancer.

Tomorrow, HOM Furniture is delivering our new couch and chair that we had made from the fabric we selected. I'm excited to see it, as it's the first quality couch and chair we've ever purchased. Flashbacks about the sales person who sold it to us keep reccurring in my mind. She shared with Jim and I about her friend who died of breast cancer. It has really made me think even more about how dangerous cancer can be. It's not something to be taken lightly. I think about her friend lying dead in her apartment with metastatic breast cancer and a hole in her body because the cancer was so aggressive. I want to cry for her and all the others who have lost loved ones to this disease.

Jim went back to school today after being off for the summer. He's glad to have a job in the mornings that he really loves. Jim truly thrives being around people, and I will have my freedom to do the things I want. He is going to physical therapy, and I give him a lot of credit for doing exercises two times a day. What a determined guy! We have a couple of potlucks at church this weekend. I wonder what I can bring that is healthy.

Pastor Joe, of Faith Lutheran Church, is coming over for a meeting with me on Thursday. I'm anxious to talk to him, as he's a man of many experiences.

How is everything going at your house? Did you hire someone to snowplow this winter? It sure worked out having someone take care of the grass and leaves for you.

138

My inner wisdom tells me that I need to be optimistic, have hope, a good attitude and positive emotions. Cancer patients need to have faith, so healing can begin. I've read that bad emotions fuel glucose or sugar in your blood. Yet, there was this Netherlands study of 9,705 women where they found emotions had no connection to cancer. We don't know all the factors that went into play. Life Extension in one of their articles stated, "Cancer has an appetite for sugar and requires sugar for survival. Sugar plays an active role in reducing immune response and energizes cancer." The article goes on to say, "There's a relationship between lactic acid, insulin, and angiogenesis. In tumors, hypoxic conditions occur through both inflammation, which reduces blood flow, and the chaotic development of blood vessels within a tumor." Isn't this interesting? I look at sweets and I think, "**Cancer!**"

Breast cancer is a wake up call to our bodies. It's important for a breast cancer patient to find out what's bothering and eating them inside. We need to treat ourselves kindly and starve the cancer, so it won't grow. I guess it's like putting poor gas and oil in the car. The car will stop running when gas is watered down, of lesser quality and it will knock . Breast cancer patients need to get their feelings out, deal with the stress head on, and forgive. Emotions, bad viruses, bacteria, fungus and cancer can cause free radials that steal your good cells away from us. Endorphins can have an effect on cancer. Once you deal with the sludge, you can forget and love one another. That's why faith, positive affirmations, mediation and yoga are helpful.

I'm going to give my worries to God tonight, so He can be in control. I have a lot of hope which I think helps my spirit. I'm putting my faith in God more than ever.

I sure wish the weather's faucet would change outside! Here are some survivor journal sheets and feeling concept sheets I made up.

Love,

Peggy

"Each one of us is someone's mother, granddaughter, aunt, friend, or soul mate. Don't let cancer defeat you." -Peggy A. Like my new quote?

Cancer Facts, Terms, Knowledge, and Concepts
<u>*Symptoms and Risk Factors:*</u>

<u>**Breast Cancer**</u>-There can be a fluctuation in estrogen and testosterone in response to depression and the inability to deal with problems. It can effect femininity, sex organs, and even create a sense of loss and grief.

<u>**Depression**</u>-Women who are depressed are four times more likely to get cancer according to a John Hopkins study.

<u>**Fatigue**</u>-To avoid fatigue stay active, exercise, sleep well, deal with the issues that bother you including depression, and anxiety. Caffeine and alcohol can effect these cycles._

<u>**Feelings**</u>- Feelings can include: grief, loss, learning to cope, vulnerability, needing emotional support, being worried, helplessness, distress, being fearful, predicting or for seeing bad outcomes, and ambivalence.

<u>**Laughter**</u>-Laughter is an important aspect of getting healthy in a cancer patient. It makes you improve your blood pressure, improve breathing, reduces hypertension, reduces your stress hormones and pain by relaxing your body, and strengthens your immune system by making you feel better about yourself.

<u>**Hope**</u>-A will to live or go on ,and is a necessary factor to improve cancer prognosis.

<u>**Stress-Anxiety-and Depression**</u>- These are products of your mind that may effect the body. They include: agitation, anger, anxiety, apprehensive, bad temper, blank thoughts, bloating feeling, blood pressure elevation, bowel problems, cold hands and feet, concentration problems, conflicts, confusion, delayed fertility and menstrual cycles, dizziness, dry mouth, eating issues, everything is in a rush, fatigue, finding fault with yourself and others, flushing skin, guilt, headaches (migraines), heart palpitations, heart burn, impotence (male), indecisiveness, increased metabolic rate, irritable, insomnia, jittery, lack of faith, life is no longer fun, money worries, muscle tension in neck, memory loss, more complaints, more illnesses, muscle tension other places in the body, nausea, nervousness, not interested in sex, overwhelmed, panic attacks, physically ill, poor blood supply, raised glucose levels, resent others who don't work, sadness, shaking, stomach aches, shortness of breath, sweating, tension, thoughts of illness and death, tiredness, trembling, unhealthy relationships, worthlessness feelings, and worrying.

<u>**Stress Stages**</u>-These stages could include alarm, resistance, and exhaustion.

<u>Diagnostic Procedures/Treatment:</u>

<u>**Happy Life**</u>- Don't be judgmental of others as they walk in different shoes. Don't seek external approval and pleasures. Live in the present and let all anger go. Listen to your body's time clock and think of positive affirmations. Get rid of toxic people and emotions. Relax. Value what is within you more and give from your heart.

<u>**How To Relax**</u>-There are many ways that you can relax. These could include breathing, counting, drinking water, finding a special spot to relax in, listening to

140

relaxing music, biofeedback, meditation, being around cool colors, writing, expressing yourself through art, reflexology, massage therapy, and going for a walk.

Stress Management:

1.Do what you can do, after you have prioritized your activities and stick to the routine.

2.Set your limits of what you can handle at home, in your family, at work, and in social activities. Also set financial limits as well.

3.Plan ahead on how you will deal with stressful situations.

4.Be positive, take a deep breath before you respond to a stressful situation, and smell life through all your senses. Relax with classes in meditation, yoga, music, other types of imagery and practice breathing everyday. Look at life with fresh eyes and a new perspective.

5.Make sure you have a survival network of friends, and learn to deal with the individual differences of the people in your life.

6.Exercise and be active.

7.Take care of your body by eating healthy, well balanced meals, skipping alcohol, stop taking sleeping pills, avoid nicotine, pop, tea, and coffee. Drink eight glasses of water a day for your cellular activity.

8.Avoid stressors and negativity. Enroll in a stress reduction class, seek help by seeing a counselor, or confide in some one close to you. Get rid of toxic people in your life that effect your emotions.

9.Sleep 7-8 hours a night.

Worry-How to stop worrying: Face the worry, deal with it by taking responsibility that you brought it on, let the obsession go, and don't waste anymore time worrying. Life is way too short.

Medical Findings from Tests/Terminology:

Hypnosis-A way to deal with pain and the bad side effects to a treatment.

Mind-Body Medicine (Psychoneuroimmunology)-This is the power that the mind has over the body's immune system, and it is a program offered at Cancer Treatment Centers of America that involves stress management, relaxation, imagery training, spiritual meditation, support groups, counseling, psycho education groups, humor therapy, and educational resources.

Mindfulness-Practicing mindfulness is paying attention to your senses as you eat, work on your posture, breathe, and work through issues by way of meditation.

Shock-A trauma to the system.

Spiritual Care-This is treatment that may involve prayer, finding a sense of meaning in life with a higher being, positive affirmations, prayer chains, spiritual counseling, worship services, healing by faith, dealing with grief through bereavement counseling, baptism, sacraments, end of life decisions, living wills, and health care directives.

Support Groups-These are groups where people can deal with decisions that have made a psychological impact on them.

Survivor's Journal

1. Traumatic events can effect your immune system by wearing it down so cancer, bacteria, and fungus can take over. Write your feelings and stressors below by putting them on the dance floor. Move your frustrations onto this paper so you don't have to dance with death.

---

2. There are always people we can't get along with, don't care for, or plain well don't like. What can you do to handle these difficult people? Write your action plan below on the clouds and let them move off into the sky.

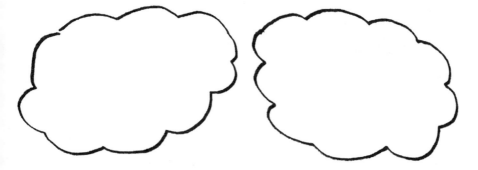

3. It's important to have a passion about things you believe in. It may even be hobbies. What hobbies do you have that bring you enjoyment? What hobbies would you like to have?

4. What makes you strong? If you were the captain of an army, how would you motivate your soldiers to fight for you? Write about your strengths on the first arrow and what you need to do to motivate your army on the second arrow.

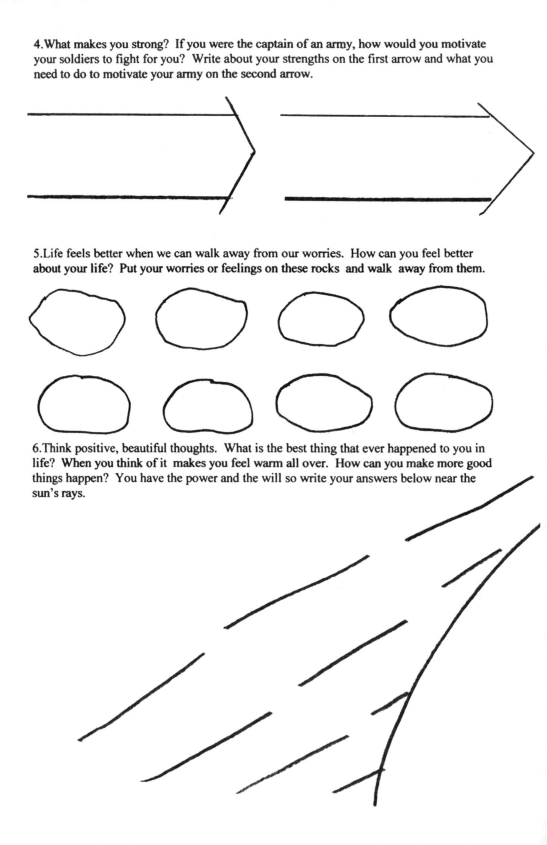

5. Life feels better when we can walk away from our worries. How can you feel better about your life? Put your worries or feelings on these rocks and walk away from them.

6. Think positive, beautiful thoughts. What is the best thing that ever happened to you in life? When you think of it makes you feel warm all over. How can you make more good things happen? You have the power and the will so write your answers below near the sun's rays.

7.Describe how you see yourself. How do you think others see you? What changes would you make? Write your answers on the people below.

Myself   **How Others See Me**   **Changes I'd Make**

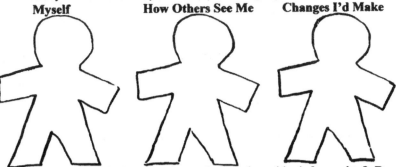

8.Describe your faith. What do you believe in and look forward to? Do you have any positive affirmations or thoughts that you live by? Write your answers below.

9.What qualities do you like best about yourself? How can you use these qualities to impact others? Your family? Your community? Your society? Write them on the smiley faces below.

Family   **Community**   **Society**

10.Goals can improve your quality of life and expectations as you seek to achieve them. What are your life goals? Goals for this year? Goals for today, this week, or month? Health goals? Relationship goals? Family goals? Financial goals? Home goals? Work goals? Write them on a separate sheet of paper.

11. Explain how you feel about having cancer. How can this learning experience help you to be more positive for your self and others? Write your answers on the cancer cells below.

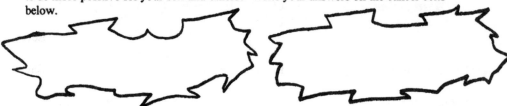

12. Explain what you have learned about BC. What do you still want to learn about BC?

13. Write your dream on the rainbow below. Direct your life to that dream.

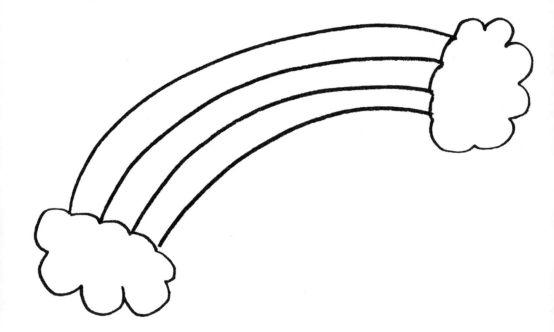

"It is a curious thing in human experience but to live through a period of stress and sorrow with another person creates a bond which nothing seems able to break."

-Eleanor Roosevelt

"The most important medicine is tender love and care." -Mother Teresa

"Things do not change, we do." -Henry David Thoreau

"Whoever sows sparingly will also reap sparingly, and whoever sows generously will also reap generously." -Corinthians 9:6

"The tongue that brings healing is a tree of life." -Proverbs 15:4

"Let no one come to you without leaving happier and better." -Mother Teresa

"Do not let any unwholesome talk come out of your mouths, but only what is helpful for building others up according to their needs, that it may benefit those who listen." -Ephesians 4:29

9/20/04

Dear Auntie,

Many of us live each day wondering what our purpose is in this game of life. I was invigorated by our chat the other night. I'm sorry you aren't feeling very well but please eat healthy.

Radiation 101 or should I say nuking is going fine except I'm a little tired. They are doing radiation in three areas. I see my doctor once a week, and a nurse as needed. My skin is a little pink but I am using Aquafor on my skin, so it doesn't get irritated. Jim enjoys coming with me to the Miller Dwan Radiation Center to chat with the other people. He says, "They have the best popcorn in town." I read books, talk a little and sometimes knit. I'm reading all their breast cancer books and watching the videos at home. It's making me think about the treatments and the causes of breast cancer. I can't believe the number of men that go there because of prostrate cancer!!! I do think Miller Dwan Hospital is the best kept secret in town!

Last week I had a CAT scan of my sinuses and teeth. My sinus passages and my mouth are really dry. I choke on my own tongue at night because my mouth is so dry.

I have no moisture anywhere, and I'm using Orajel, a toothpaste, for dry mouth and Biotene gum for my salvia problems. I can't get those salvia tablets you gave me for my mouth at Plaza Walgreens. Radiation, hot flashes and hormone blocking can cause a person to have salvia problems, and it sure dries you out. Drinking a whole lot more water should be top priority for me. Unfortunately, I'm not very hungry or thirsty, and I feel like I've been living on the desert.

I'm so glad that you're praying for me. I always knew I had guardian angels, and you sure make a special angel. There are angels in all of us if we search for them and help each other. I do trust God's choices and His sovereignty. Attitude is important for a cancer patient and faith.

Life is good. I have my senior driver's class the next two nights. This is the class to get a reduction on my insurance as well as a refresher class for those who are over 55. I'm not looking forward to being there so long because I keep getting bad hot flashes all the time. They would die in class if I started my Lady Godiva act of taking my top clothes off. I wish I knew the answer on how to stop these hot flashes dead in their tracks.

I have a meeting with Kim Lakhen, my vivacious ENT physician assistant, at the clinic tomorrow to go over my CAT scan. It's very early, but then we are nocturnal people.

That's all. Tell me a little more about Grandma and her breast cancer sometime.

Love,

Peggy

September 30, 2004

Dear Peggy,

Your phone call last week about your radiation treatments reminded me of when Mom had undergone radiation at St. Luke's Hospital. This was after our return from the Mayo Clinic in 1952. Earlier this spring, I wrote you about Mom's cancer experience in 1936.

After that March 7, 1952 appointment with the internal medicine physician, she came over to the insurance office where I worked as an office manager. She was very pale and told me she didn't know what to do, as the doctor had told her that she had metastasized cancer, and he couldn't help her. The doctor confirmed the diagnosis when I called him. While I was talking to him, I asked about taking her to the Mayo for a second opinion. He agreed and offered to make arrangements for her to be admitted as an inpatient, so there wouldn't be a delay.

Dad drove us down to Rochester. We got Mom checked in at the Methodist Hospital, and I got checked into the nearby Kahler Hotel. When we checked Mom in, we were told of a trial study underway regarding the use of a "radioactive iodine cocktail" to aid in locating cancers. If we agreed that upon her death, we would have an autopsy done, a copy sent to them, and there would be no charge for this procedure. Dad left for home. He said, "for business," but in truth, he couldn't handle his concern.

The day of the "cocktail" test Mom was placed under a machine that went over her body slowly, section by section. As the machine kept clicking away, Mom asked me, if I thought the clicks indicated that her cancer was in that many places. I remember telling her, "That maybe that's just what the machine does." When the doctors made their rounds that evening, they signaled me out into the hall. They said that the next day they would be discharging Mom and having a meeting with her regarding her serious condition. The answer to my question of "how long?" put me out cold on the floor. I had fainted when told in their judgment, three or four months.

Now remember, I thought her appointment a few days earlier in Duluth was a routine check up. As soon as I got back to the hotel I called Dad. We both agreed that we did not want Mom hit with this terrible news so fast. Today we know better, patients are entitled to be fully aware of their condition, and a partner in all decisions, but everything was happening so fast.

Dad drove down early the next morning and arranged to meet with one of the doctors before their meeting with Mom. Dad was adamant that she was not to be told how dire her situation was. Mayo would not deceive their patient. But Dad, the #1 salesman of the world's largest wholesale hardware company, Marshall Wells, could be very persuasive and firm. A compromise was reached. They would not go into full detail of her terminal cancer, unless they were asked. The doctors would suggest radiation as that might delay the end. But they told Dad, it was too late to rid her body of cancer.

On our drive home later that day, Mom was pretty quiet, until she asked us, "Why don't they just operate?" I answered by telling her, "That is something we could think about if the radiation doesn't help." I said, "think," I knew the answer. We were trying to delay her knowledge. To all outward appearances she wasn't sick, had never mentioned or complained about any troubles, and was very active in life. Earlier that winter, Mom and I had been on a tour of many tourist places in Florida. She had her radiation that spring and by summer was back on the golf course.

Mom and I returned to Florida for a month that next winter. During the summer her numerous hospital trips and various health complications started. Dad died (October 9, 1953), from a heart attack en route to the hospital. I have always believed from "a broken heart." All those worries he had for so many years were finally happening. After Dad's death, I quit working to care for Mom. I had realized before that the time was coming where she needed more help.

After Christmas in January 1954, we drove south for the winter. Traveling was very hard for Mom, but after a few days in the sun she would rally. We would spend our days at the pool or on the ocean beach front. She enjoyed going to the horse races, dog tracks or park concerts. Her strength was limited but she had great determination to enjoy each day of her life.

That summer Mom had an emergency tracheotomy while in the hospital for some other cancer related problem. The tissue surrounding the tube wouldn't heal properly and required frequent use of a suction machine. From that time on, whenever she was hospitalized, I stayed with her. I was now on 24 hour, seven days a week duty, with very few exceptions. After Mom's trach, climbing stairs became a problem. We moved to a bungalow on Vermillion Road. She no longer wanted company to come over, she never wanted anyone to "pity her."

The snow was falling that January morning in Duluth of '55 as we once again headed for Florida's sun. It was a long trip as she had to be hospitalized in Kentucky, and we needed to stop often to keep her trach tube open. Mom usually wore a light chiffon neckerchief over the tube and to speak she would have to cover the tube opening.

Mom's hair by now was a beautiful platinum color, she was very thin, very fragile and would tire easily. The sun again did the job. Our days were quiet, she did less, but a good part of the day was spent in the sun. Usually, sitting by the pool while I read a book on a water float. We'd often go to the town park concerts, and we headed home in spring.

All this writing about how the sun would invigorate Mom makes me wonder. She had spent years on the golf course, seldom used any tanning lotion, would never burn, but never got dark as I would. Now we are warned about using the right protective covering. Can this be from environmental changes?

In the summer Mom started to have trouble swallowing and had to have a stomach tube put in for feeding. I learned in a hurry how to feed her, as well as how to inject her morphine. Our very close friends, Evelyn and Bill Annand, either stopped by each day or called to check on how things were going. Evelyn was the Assistant Director of Nursing at St. Lukes Hospital and would hook up her IV's when needed, as well as handle the muscle injections. We made a good hospice team. Without her help, Mom couldn't have stayed at home. Evelyn, who had been such an angel to Mom, died in 1962, at the age of 40 of an aneurism. As ill as Mom was, every time she had to go to the hospital, she would remark, "how thankful she was and how sorry she felt for all those sick people." In my nightly prayers, I always asked God, that there would be something good for her the next day, and that when the time came for Him to take her from us, it would be quick, without further pain.

On Mom's 56th birthday, November 21,st she told me, as she had several times before, that she thought it was time for her to go. As I always did, I told her that suitcase was getting all worn out from all those trips she didn't take. This time she didn't budge. From time to time she would mention to me, with the changing of the seasons, what she wanted to wear for her funeral. We never dwelt on the subject of death, it would be said off hand.

Three days later, on Thanksgiving, she wouldn't let me give her any pain medication until I had my Thanksgiving dinner. She didn't want me to eat that holiday meal alone, and was concerned that she might doze off. I ate my TV turkey dinner in her bedroom. One week after her last birthday she was gone, November 28, 1955.

During the last months there were many nights of her pacing the floor repeating the Twenty-third Psalm. I worried that I might not hear her in the night if she needed me, and I had your dad put a doorbell by her bed to my headboard. For the first time in my adult life, I climbed into her single bed with her to sleep on the 27,th in case she needed oxygen, which was now on standby. When I woke up, she was gone. I have always appreciated that I had spent that night next to her, I knew her death was peaceful. The power of prayer is great, that's just how it happened.

Those last years of Mom's life were hard. But with the help of good friends, good doctors that would come to our home whenever needed, and Zion Lutheran Church minister's weekly visits to give her communion, it was bearable. Mom's good spirits, her enjoyment of life, even as her ability to participate would lessen, and her strong faith in God kept her going. She had reached acceptance about her illness, had no fear of dying, but kept on trying to do her best in life. I have always been thankful that I had the opportunity to be by her side on her final journey. I was in an unique position, I didn't have to work for income, I was still single, my only responsibility and desire were caring for her.

Writing this letter brings up so many sad memories, but also reconfirms my belief that through prayer, much strength can be received to handle difficult times. Those sixteen years of remission for no known cause after unsuccessful surgery, no chemo, or radiation, little or no doctoring from 1936 to 1952 have always raised a question within me. Was it her determination and faith in God? An answer to her prayers? Or what?

Peggy, I hope the experiences of your Grandmother Prahl from fifty years ago, give you courage to never give up hope. Your part is to give your best efforts through the guidance of your doctors and prayers. Don't sit back and wait for the next crisis. Don't miss any cancer appointments, see the doctor when you see any suspicious signs, be ready to start chemo if necessary, and continue researching about cancer. I want you to take good care of your health and conquer your disease. There are many more years ahead of you.

Love always,

Aunt Karen

152

P.S. On Tuesday, I took Jim to the doctor as he was having trouble breathing and his body was so swollen. Turns out he was suffering from 'heart failure." The increase in his diuretics is getting rid of all the extra fluid, and the cardiogram didn't show any new damage to his heart. The twins made their first visit here that night to check on Grandpa!

"We began by imagining that we are giving to them; we end by realizing that they have enriched us."   -Pope John Paul II

"For I know the plans I have for you," declares the Lord. "Plans to prosper you and not to harm you, plans to give you hope and a future."   -Jeremiah 29

"I have found that four faiths are crucial to recovery from serious illness: faith in oneself, one's doctor, one's treatment, and one's spiritual faith."   -Bernie Siegel MD

"Sorrow looks back, worry looks around, faith looks up."   -Ralph Waldo Emerson

"Love the Lord, your God with all your heart and all your soul and with your mind and with all your strength."   -Mark 12:30

"Give yourself to God…Surrender your whole being to him to be used for righteous purposes."   -Roman 6:13

10/1/04

Dear Auntie,

Five days out of the week I go to my daily ritual of radiation. The staff are so kind, gregarious and sensitive to the patients. In fact, they are very humorous at times. I tell them this place should be called "Miller Dwan Med" after Club Med because patients get partially naked from the waist up. It reminds me of one of our two French exchange students who came from a family of two doctors. This particular student would go with her mom to sun bathe topless at Club Med on holidays.

Oh, one of the technicians has had breast cancer. I think I'll give her a little gift at the end because she's extra kind to me. I'm knitting a breast cancer pink hat and scarf for Dr. Park Skinner, and two technicians wanted the pattern. We're not suppose to diet, but maintain our weight. In fact, we need to eat more calories during radiation. The first day I got a list of types of food I should eat. I don't want my body's immune system to be tricked by the enemy, so I'll have to follow their directives.

Some strange things have been happening with my health. As I told you before my eyes, mouth, and throat are extremely dry, as are other body parts. I saw Dr. Skorich, my exuberant eye doctor, on the 24th and he gave me a prescription for some eye drops called Restasis to help my severe dry eye condition. The doc said he could put plugs in my tear drains (ducts), if this doesn't work.

I saw Kim Lakhen, my knowledgeable ENT physician assistant, about my CAT scan on the 21st, and she wants me to see my dentist, Dr. Bussa. I have a split up my tooth down to the root and a cyst. Dr. Bussa, whose very perceptive, referred me to Dr. Kronzer. Kim Lakhen also recommended that I buy a one quart container at Target to carry around with me. That's how much water she wants me to drink a day as I'm so dried out. My nasal passages and mouth are very dry. I know it's from lack of hormones, but maybe some from radiation. I'm trying to drink up the lake now.

Not to go on a bird walk about radiation, but one woman at support group told us that she cried and cried at radiation years ago because she didn't understand the whole procedure. Fear can be a powerful factor.

Yesterday I had my appointment with Dr. Windberg, the sleep apnea doctor at the Duluth Clinic, and he feels I don't have sleep apnea. He told me why and gave me suggestions on what I can do to sleep better. Not sleeping is a part of my life right now. He thinks I will go back to my normal pattern at some point.

Love,

Peggy

Dale Carnegie--"You have it easily in your power to increase this world's happiness now. How? By giving a few words of sincere appreciation to someone who is lonely or discouraged. Perhaps you will forget tomorrow the kind words you say today, but the recipient may cherish them over a life time.

Cancer Facts, Terms, Knowledge and Concepts

Symptoms:
Aromatase Inhibitors-These are androstenodine drugs that block estrogen.
Asomasin Side Effects-Side effects may include cough, chills, fever, hoarseness, low back and side pain, increased blood pressure, shortness of breathe, swelling of hands, legs and feet.
Excessive Estrogen-From excessive estrogen you may have longer periods, irregular periods, dense breasts, breast disease, breast and uterine cancer, and endometriosis.
Femara Side Effects-Side effects may include shortness of breath.
Hormone Therapy-There are many drugs to block estrogen. They include Tamoxifen, Goserlin (Zoladex) and aromatase inhibitors as Armidex, Leptosome (Femera), and Exemestane (Aromasin).
Lack of Estrogen-If you don't have enough estrogen you can stop having your periods, get osteopenia, osteoporosis, go into early menopause, become infertile, have hot flashes, have vaginal burning, and may have skin irritation from sexual activity.
Menopause Symptoms and a Need for Hormone Therapy: These may include depression, fatigue, headache, heart disease, hot flashes, insomnia, loss of bladder control, loss of sex drive, memory loss, night sweats, osteoporosis, vaginal dryness, and weight gain.
Osteoporosis-This is when the bone deteriorates leading to brittleness. A person can have increased risk of broken bones and a hump can develop on the back.
Serious Side Effects of Hormone Therapy: These may include blood clots, change in vision, infections, infections, inflammation of the throat, painful joints and muscles, rash, shortness of breath, sinus trouble, and upset stomach.
Tamoxifen Side Effects-Patients can get back pain, blood clots, hair loss, fatigue, hot flashes and nausea.

Diagnostic Procedures/ Treatments:
Bone Density Test-A test that measures how dense and strong your bones are, compares it to other tests, measures bone loss, and helps to determine treatments that should be done.
DEXA(Dual Energy X-ray/Absorptiometry Scan)-This test measures calcium in the bones.
Estrogen Imbalance: Excessive Estrogen can show up as very dense breasts or proliferate breast disease, breast cancer, uterine cancer, endometriosis, irregular or excessive menses. **Lack of Estrogen** can show up as hot flashes, vaginal dryness, osteoporosis, ending of menses, infertility, and premature menopause.
High Risk Post Menopausal Women-Some sources feel that these women should not do hormone therapy. They should avoid alcohol or drink very little.
Hormones-These are natural chemicals found in your body that regulate processes as

bone growth, milk production in the breasts, and blood sugar metabolism. Some types of hormones are insulin, estrogen, and adrenaline.

Hormonal Profile Range (Normal for Women)-(From Life Extension)-
Estradiol (<5.0-54.72 pg/mL)
Progesterone (0.1-0.8ng/mL)
Testosterone Total (6.0-82 ng/dL); Free (0.03-1.55 pg/mL)
Follicle Stimulating Hormone (FSH) (25.8-134.8 mIU/mL)
Luteinizing Hormone (LH) (7.7-58.5 mIU/mL)
DHEA-S (10-190 ug/dL)

HRT (Hormone Replacement Therapy)- Hormones are used to restore the estrogen by the ovaries. HRT is often used to prevent fractures, prevent osteoporosis, heart attacks, heart disease, reduce the side effects of menopause and help other parts of the body to function effectively. Hormone pills are usually taken once a day to help women with the onset of menopause as they get older. Progesterone often declines as women get older. (Women do gain weight from HRT pills.)

Laparoscope-This is the removing of the ovaries through incisions in the abdomen. If you do this, it drops your cancer risk by 50%. You can still get cancer in the same place after removal.

Ovarian Suppression-The patient is given hormone blocker medicine to shut down the ovaries. An example is Zoladex. It may help to remove the ovaries and having low dose radiation in this area.

Medical Findings/Terminology:

Agonist-This would keep a woman from not getting the bad effects of estrogen loss as good bone density.

Aldosterone-A steroid that acts in the kidneys to control your sodium balance in the body.

Calcium D-Glucrate-A brand name calcium that helps with major detoxification of the pathways in the body as well as liver excretion of estrogen.

Cortisol-This is a steroid involved in immune functions in the body.

EDG1(Estrogen-Regulated Gene 1)-A gene that is found to be switched off by estrogen when there is increased breast cancer growth. When this gene is over expressed there will be a decrease in cell growth and support.

Estradiol-A hormone produced by the ovaries, adrenal glands, and peripheral tissues. It is an indicator of pituitary and hypothalamic function. It can have an effect on bone density.

Estrogen-A female sex hormone produced mostly by the ovaries. Progesterone is also produced by the ovaries. Estrogen is made during the entire menstrual cycle. Women are never without estrogen because it continues to be made by the glands and the body fat. It is needed by other body organs as well. Estrogen improves your mental state and lowers your bodies blood sugars. It's an important key to your receptors. Estrogen tells the alpha receptors to let estrogen in and the beta receptors to keep it out. When estrogen falls during menopause hot flashes decline.

Estrogen Dominance-When you are estrogen dominant it can causes breast cancer. Other causes could include an under active thyroid, excessive phytoestrogens, exposure to pesticides or ingestion of pesticides. There are side effects from too much estrogen and they include: thrombosis, embolism, stroke, hypoxia, edema, heart attack, seizures, migraines, hypoglycemia, and fluid retention.

Estrogen-Progesterone Balance-You need balance in your body. Estrogen circulates though out your body, is produced in the body, and binds to receptors (alpha and beta). Estrogen is broken down and eliminated in the body as well.

Estrone-This is a hormone produced in the fatty tissue of the body.

Fat Cells-Fat cells produce small amounts of estrogen. After menopause estrogen is produced in the fat cells as the ovaries shut down. This is the reason why obese and post menopausal women are more at risk in breast cancer prognosis.

Hormone Blockers-These drugs include Tamoxifen (Nolvadex), Raloxifene, Toremifene (Fareston) and aromatase inhibitors (Armidex).

Letrozole-A hormone blocker that stops estrogen.

Lupron (Leuprolide)-This is a drug that blocks the ovaries from functioning.

LHRH (Lutenizing Hormone-Release Agonists)-These are drugs that keep the ovaries from working. They include Zoladex (Goserlin), Lupron, and Triptorelin (Trelstar Depot).

Progesterone-Another name for a hormone produced by the ovaries and responsible for menstrual cycles.

Menopause-This is when your body stops producing hormones. Often this occurs at ages 40-50 and you begin your change of life.

NSAIDS (Nonsteroidal Anti-inflammatory) Drugs-These can reduce inflammation in the breast tissue and prevent cancer.

Ovaries-Ovaries before menopause produce most of the estrogen in women's bodies.

Progesterone-This female hormone is produced in the ovaries during the second half of the menstrual cycle to prepare for fertilization. It can be converted to cortical and testosterone. Too much progesterone can be a downer. It can bring on fatigue and depression. It can also raise sugar levels, balance estrogen, protect against fibrocystic heart disease, restore sex drive, prevents breast cancer, balances cortical levels, helps to prevent osteoporosis and bone loss.

Progestin-This is a synthetic form of progesterone similar to that which is produced in the body.

Tamoxifen-Anti estrogen blocker drug for estrogen positive women who are pre menopausal to ward off breast cancer. Several studies have shown that " 30% of patients acquire Tamoxifen resistance and relapse into the disease," according to Medscape. After using this drug there is strong evidence that women are at high risk for getting uterine, gastrointestinal and fatal liver cancer.

Testosterone-Women have this sex hormone in their bodies but at a lesser amount that men. It helps with muscle strength, bone mass, and sexual function.

Triglycerides-These fluctuate from excessive refined sugars, alcohol, and starches.

Estrogen Fits Into The Receptors And Promotes Cell Division

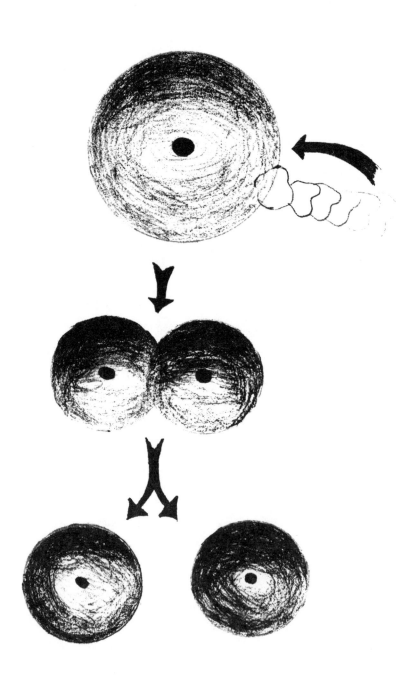

"Adversity is not without comforts and hopes."   -Francis Bacon

"God sometimes puts us on our back, so that we may look upward.
                                                            -Unknown Author

"Every moment of time holds a gift in its hands."   -Unknown Author

"But those who hope in the Lord will renew their strength. They will soar on wings like eagles; they will run and grow weary, they will walk and not be faint."   -Isaiah 40:31

"My soul finds rest in God alone; my salvation comes from him."   -Psalm 62:1

"In all your ways acknowledge him, and he will make your paths straight."
                                                            -Proverbs 3:6

10/31/04

Dear Auntie,

    Here's a few quick pictures of what's been going on in my photo album. Radiation ended on October 21st. After radiation, I have a follow up appointment in November with Dr. Frye. My underarm and breast are not looking too good, and he gave me a big jar of Silvadene with gauze. Going to radiation has been a part of my life five days a week, for at least seven weeks. I do get pretty tired but the staff are really great about cheering everyone up.

    Did I tell you that Dr. Frye said they identified a protein in women with high risk for breast cancer? I should of asked him what it was called. Now my thoughts will wonder off with the clouds about this protein.

    I wanted to tell you that I received some gifts from Miller Dwan Radiation for breast cancer awareness: a pin, a cup, and sticky notes from the technicians, nurses, and doctors. They are very special! I brought some healthy cakes a week before for the staff, and fresh fruit in a fall basket my last week with T-shirts that Jim and I made for them. We put the lettering, "October is Breast Cancer Awareness Month" on the shirts with a breast cancer symbol. The staff took a few pictures of us wearing the shirts. They gave me a couple of copies of the picture and a certificate. They will always hold a special place in my heart.

Backtracking on Oct. 8th, I had to be re-measured for radiotherapy super boosts to my lumpectomy spot as well as my the auxiliary area. This was simpler and was for the last seven days of treatment. It took less time.

The good news, bad news in review is a summary of my breast cancer. You were wondering about my final diagnosis on the last report. I want to clarify my final diagnosis of breast and lymph cancer. The type was infiltrating ductual carcinoma in the left breast, the grade was intermediate grade and the stage was IIA. I also had another type called DCIS. It seems the forms were called comedo and crib. I had three surgeries for a lumpectomy to get clear margins and auxiliary node dissection. The primary tumor was 1.5 in the left breast. I've had 21 nodes removed, one with cancer. The secondary tumor in the node was 2.5 grossly and 2 cm microscopically because there was focal vascular invasion in the soft perinodal tissue. My tumor was ER (estrogen) and PR (progesterone) positive. My primary tumor was tested for HER/neu and was HER/neu 2 plus. It was sent away to be tested by the FISH test as well.

Besides the three surgeries, I had radiation and now I'm on this estrogen blocking drug, Armidex. Supposedly, this drug is for post menopausal women with mestastic breast disease. I read on the internet that you need to take calcium when on Armidex. My Blue Cross-Blue Shield case manger sent me a sheet from the internet about complementary therapies. One fact stated that Calcium D Glucarate is good because it detoxifies the excessive estrogen from the liver. I wonder where you get this particular calcium. Maybe I need a bone density test in the future. Armidex can eliminate a few hot flashes, cause diarrhea, and may cause bone density problems. It's a drug that may have other uses in the future.

Thinking about my choices, I did have a choice to have my breast removed. In fact, I could have had both breasts removed because of my strong family history of breast cancer and the metastitic invasive part of the problem. I just couldn't handle it at this point in time, and I wanted the least invasive procedure. The reccurrence is very much the same. Maybe it is slightly more. This plan may not be the best for most women, because it depends on many, many factors. It depends on the type of cancer, the stage, the grade, and the metastasis. Any choice you make needs to be made with qualified doctor recommendations.

You know, I had a choice and chose not to do chemo. The reason for not doing it at this time was that it only increased my chances by a few percentage points. I have other medical issues, and I would do it in the future if necessary. There are shadows of concern over the tumor I had under my arm. But I have had radiation in the breast and under the arm. My chances are real good, I think, I hope, I pray.

As a patient, I think it's important to look at all the possible causes of my breast cancer and make changes in those areas to prevent reccurrences. If a reccurrence happens, it's not my doctors fault. A few cells could have strayed away. I need to find the cause of my cancer and try to prevent it, so I don't get cancer again.

I had to go to the chiropractor on Oct. 5th as my neck hurt from lying on the linear accelerator machine as I have neck problems anyway. I do miss Dr. Ladd but Dr. Torgrimson was my chiropractor many, many years ago, and he's really super. I told him a cool idea for a T-shirt next year. It was a skeleton on a black shirt with the letters "Keep your Skelton Straight." He laughed and jokingly said, "I should hire you for advertising." On the night of the 5th, I had to go to Miller Dwan for radiation. Those technicians sure work long hours.

Lots has been happening around here. "The Anderson Twins," as Annie calls them, went for their haircuts at Amity Kennels. We call her Aunt Annie at home when we tell our dogs they are going for hair cuts or to be boarded. Annie loves dogs in spite of being allergic to them. They sure become cranky dogs after their haircuts.

Life continues onward and we are as busy as ever. Bible Study is Thursday. Jim had FEMA practice on the 16th which was very interesting. We helped with the church carnival after I baked a few more cakes. On the 26th I went to a tasting party at Helen's called *Tastefully Simple*. I had my hair colored the same day, and you wouldn't recognize me. Saturday night we went to a movie at church. Then came Halloween and we didn't have many trick or treaters. I didn't dress up the dogs this year either. Jim is so busy with so many activities that it enriches his life as well as the community.

We were overjoyed to see you on the 8th. The Red Roof Inn was comfortable and was free with our points. We did miss the Woodland Community Bazaar by coming back late on Saturday. I had also wanted to go to some knitting demonstration at the mall which I didn't make it to. There are only so many moments in time, and I try to balance everything in my life.

I went on Oct. 11th to see Dr. Seidelmann after being referred by Dr. Kronzer. They both very conscientious dentists. It was interesting having a Panorex x-ray. Then on the 20th I had oral surgery on my tooth. I go back to see Dr. Seidelmann in March for another test. This was the day that the Central Retirees went to the Boathouse for lunch, and I couldn't go. What a busy life being retired. I'm running too much.

Life continues on. I saw Dr. Bloom, gynecologist at the Duluth Clinic on the 22nd because of my dry conditions. He is very upbeat and spontaneous. On the 29th I went for some free testing on peripheral vascular disease for the "Legs for Life" screening program which also involved an ultrasound. It's great that the clinic has this program. I told a friend about it at the clinic one day, and she asked me how I found out about it. I said, "It was in the Duluth News-Tribune. I signed up for it this summer, and it was free! I was on a waiting list as so many signed up." I couldn't get Jim to sign up.

This summer Lisa would bring me flowers from the St. Paul Farmer's Market, and I really relished them. Since then I have bought flowers and given them to people with my estate sale vases. I love the look of a single carnation in a long tall vase. We all need to do special things for ourselves as life is so short. We need to appreciate all that there is in nature, go for walks and live life with full exhalation.

You asked me on the phone to think about my stressors. Well, I think we all live to make money which is the root of all evil, but a necessary substance. (Jim says it is the root of survival.) Unfortunately, we need it to live on while we try to spend our lives trying to create a worthwhile life full of meaning.

I think teachers are a different breed because we are very holistic people who search for the whole picture with our very educated mentalities. We are lovers of reading, writing, curriculum and teaching. As professional students we are lovers of the verbal and non-verbal attributes in life. Teachers value all of society including those possessions of beauty and intelligence. We try to organize, store, regurgitate information to the whole point of being eccentric and electric at times. Our decisions are based on facts after looking at the whole scheme of things. At times we want everyone else to get with the rest of the program.

My life as a teacher has been seasoned with time. I am a person who can self motivate myself. I'm a product of many experiences and proud of those experiences. I've tried to weave my memories into my daily living. I can feel pain because of past deaths that I've dealt with in my life. Deaths haunt me about students and family members who have died, those who have lost their lives to car accidents, murder and suicide. I've had to heal emotionally on my own. Death sure walks in many types of footsteps. We have to learn how to live with grief, go through the process and go forward.

I guess Auntie, we are all authors or writers of our own lives. We make our own stories. God surely has given us a purpose in this life. If we let Him, he can put his spirit in our mind and our bodies. When we do so, we add spiritual healing to our resources, to make us more resilient to diseases that effect the body. I read somewhere that faith and attitude effect a cancer patients outcome as well as strength to overcome the difficulties along the way. I think faith gives us a sense of peace, a sense of purpose, a mission in life, and an action plan for our lives. What do you think? Call me.

I leave for my trip on the 12th of November.

Love,

Peggy

"Time wasted can never be recovered; no man ever possessed the same moment twice."
-Author Unknown

"That man is truly wise who gains his wisdom from the experience of another."
-Platus

"The invariable mark of wisdom is to see the miraculous in the common."
-Ralph Waldo Emerson

"You have made known to me the path of life."   -Psalm 16:11

"Love covers all wrongs."   -Proverbs 10:12

11/26/04

Dear Auntie,

Greetings and salutations! I thought I'd write you with some more details about my trip, since I couldn't explain it all on the phone.

This really was a "celebration of life trip" for me and much more than I expected. I've learned that you need to celebrate life each day as it will never be the same again. Kay and I met at the George Bush Airport in Houston with excited anticipation. From there we took a limo to the Galveston Hilton. Wow, that was a great hotel with a view of the Gulf of Mexico and beautiful first class rooms. That night we had a superb seafood dinner at Landry's Seafood House.

The next day we embarked from Galveston on the Celebrity ship called *Galaxy*. We were out to sea for a day before arriving in Cozumel, Mexico, which was laced with white sand and very turquoise waters. I experienced a bad headache from carrying one piece of luggage at the airport. Consequently, while on the ship we decided to have full body massages. It helped my headache somewhat. In Cozumel we went by an air-conditioned bus to visit Mayan structures on the island. We went to Cedral, the oldest settlement on the island. Then we went shopping and had a light lunch. Since we couldn't complete my dream of horse back riding on the beach due to my arm and Kay's knee, we did the next best thing. I asked Kay, half laughing, "Do you want your picture taken with a donkey since we can't go horseback riding?" She said, "Sure, after I look in this black coral shop." Well, I had my picture taken next to the donkey and Kay decided to try to mount hers. She hurt her leg and hip. So much for mounting donkeys in Cozumel!

That night on the ship we went to one of George Solomon's shows. He's a singer and performer from Las Vegas. He came and sat on Kay's lap few times, and I swear she wasn't going to let him off. We more than chuckled at that as we drank our Long Island teas. After this we cruised on to Costa Maya, Mexico. The waters still remained turquoise and sand was white. The shopping was superb.

Then we were back to sea again and entered the Panama Cruising Canal. This is where Kay and I went to the Embera Indian Village by boat. We had to take the Changres River through the rain forest to Gatun Lake. The Embera Indians live much like they did a hundred years ago with a rich culture of traditions. They can't survive off the land, so they sell crafts to earn money to buy basic necessities that can't be grown. The Embera danced for us, we brought their crafts and visited their living quarters. They live up in thatched trees and their bedrooms are separated by sheets for family privacy. The women wear nothing on the top or may have a necklace fully laden with very antique coins, and they don't realize the value of these coins. Interesting enough, no one has a breast removed. Women wear colorful skirt wraps, whereas the men wore a pair of shorts with a long colorful flap in the front, past their knees. We were invited to dance with them at the end of the performance. One man's eyes bulged when he was asked to dance with a very well, overly indulged, topless girl. We returned by boat to Cristobal Pier after drinking bottled water.

After this we cruised into the Panama Locks, Kay's dream vacation, which was very exciting. In the middle of the night we were up taking pictures of the locks as we went through them at 5:00 a.m. Who wouldn't be excited at this once in a lifetime experience?

From the Canal, we went to Puerto Limon, Costa Rica. This was a trip to view the local native habitat, flora and fauna, as well as see the tropical rain forest. We learned that the guide had contracted the deadly yellow fever. She explained that the second time she would get it, she would will bleed to death. I know I DIDN'T want to go into the rainforest. When I saw a few insects flying around our boat I moved and was thankful I used my DEET spray. I had also been instructed by the Duluth Clinic Travel Center to not wear pink. After the canal trip, we went for a quick tropical fruit buffet and shopping of local crafts. We didn't realize until later we had been in an area that had a substantial earthquake a day earlier. I guess all life has risks.

After a day at sea with numerous activities we arrived at our next port of call which was Montego Bay, Jamaica. The sandy white beaches and thatched roofed huts on the beaches will remain engraved in my memory. This was a port that Kay had stayed with her family for two weeks. She really liked it and it really appealed to me as well. The tour of Jamaica included the Three Palm Golf Course and Historic Rose Hall. We wished Kay's husband, Dick, was there. This famous golf course is known because Annie Palmer, who was called the "White Witch of Rose Hall," killed three of her husbands and buried them under three palm trees. She practiced voodoo and even killed her boyfriend's daughter who later killed her. After this we went shopping at Half Moon shopping mall, then went to Aqua Sol Beach for drinks and listened to Reggae Music. I wished I had bought some of the cool clothes. Tourists are only allowed on certain beaches.

That night there was a deck party on the ship and I fell fast asleep. Michelle took my picture while I was sleeping. She wondered how anyone could sleep amidst all the deck activity.

Next stop on the cruise itinerary was Georgetown, Grand Cayman. This is where Pastor Joe has a brother living on a turtle farm. The scenery brought to mind John Grishman's best seller novels, *The Pelican Brief* and *The Firm*. We went on a glass bottom boat and took pictures of the fish swimming in the Caribbean blue waters, continued shopping all over and visited a very famous black coral shop. Kay is wild over rare black coral. I can't see how this town is damaged from the terrible hurricanes, but then I have nothing to compare it to. Grand Cayman is quite the hot spot.

We were back at sea for two more days before getting back to Galveston. I'll always remember the high tea, the afternoon teas at 4:00 p.m., the Hawaiian Lula, Kay's beehive hat, the wealth of stories about traveling from senior citizens, George Solomon, and our pictures. My picture on the bulletin board for best single model will remain with me forever.

The energetic staff on the cruise treated us superbly well by being so polite and kind. The shows were very good, some better than others, some exceptional. Kay was in the talent show as Gerry and Edna were, who sat at our table each night along with John and Michelle. They were the best company ever, as well as regular all time cruisers. I loved the exquisite food, and there were a plenty of healthy choices to choose from. Food that would detoxify, seafood and fish choices is what I ate. They had a sushi bar also. I only gained a pound because the last five days I walked three miles a day at 5:00 a.m. on the upper deck. My arm seemed a little swollen, and I wished I would of known that I should of worn the compression sleeve .

You may wonder about the waves and if we could feel them. At times the waves were very strong due to the weather. The stabilizers weren't always on, probably because of the price of fuel, and there was an earthquake. At times I'd joke, " I feel like a milk shake." The funniest story came from Gerry when he said, " I got up in the middle of night and fell on top of Edna because of the waves." The advantage of a smaller ship is that it can fit through the Panama Canal.

The trip was so great. I got a chance to meet wonderful people, walk a lot, enjoy the warmth of the sun and gulf breezes. It made me decide I want a better life style. By that I mean eating better and exercising more. Taking time to breathe more oxygen and drinking more water to flush my system of the impurities. The people were all so wonderful. I know life is great because of the people I know and meet.

This is a little radiation humor for you. I wrote a card to Dr. Frye because I was specifically told not to sunbathe. I found that there was a topless bathing on the fourteenth deck, so I wrote him and said, " I thought I'd go sunbathing, on the topless deck or buy a coconut shell bra in Jamaica to use for sunbathing, but I remembered what you said." I didn't get to mail the card until I got back. He probably got a few laughs, which was my plan.

This ends my tale of the trip with my "diamond of the desert sister-in-law." Kay sure loves diamonds, but I wonder if she knows they are made of coal?

Love,

Peggy

I'll always remember our wonderful trip but especially the sunsets and sunrises. There is much to savor in my upstairs attic. I'll remember that there are healthy choices of food which are important for the immune system. Our bodies need over 50 recognized nutrients. We all need to have a good quality palatable life. People need to be sold on themselves, so they can achieve a quality life and living. Attitude, optimism, hope, effort, courage, and determination are important in this cancer fight and mystery of life. I want to be a winner, so I don't look behind, but look ahead and remember each moment.

Some Positive Affirmations

Attitude- "The longer I live, the more I realize the impact of attitude on life. Attitude, to me, is more important than facts. It is more important than the past, than education, than money, than circumstances, than failures, than successes, than what other people think or say or do. It is more important than appearance, giftedness, or skill. It can make or break a company...a church...a home. The remarkable thing is we have a choice every day regarding the attitude we will embrace for that day. We cannot change our past...we cannot change the fact that people will act in a certain way. We cannot change the inevitable. The only thing we can do is play on the one thing we have, and that is attitude…I am convinced that life is 10% what happens to me and 90% how I react to it. And so it is with you…we are in charge of our Attitudes."

-Charles Swindoll

"YOU CAN'T CHOOSE YOUR CIRCUMSTANCES, BUT YOU CAN CHOOSE TO OVERCOME THEM."   -Author Unknown

"Twelve Steps to Vitality: 1.Whisper Good Thoughts 2.Pace Yourself 3.Think Positively 4.Go With Strengths 5.Treat Your Body Kindly 6.Nourish Spirituality 7.Cultivate Positive Friends 8.Pick Fights Carefully 9.Learn To Let Go 10.Celebrate 11.Continue to Grow 13. Find Humor"   -Dr. Tom Boman, UMD

People who know how to brighten a day with heartwarming smiles and with kind words they say, People who know how to willingly share, who know how to give and know how to care, who know how to let all their warm feelings show.. Are people that others feel lucky to know.   -Amanda Bradley

"Since the mind is a specific biocomputer, it needs specific instructions and directions. The reason most people never reach their goals is that they don't define them, learn about them, or ever seriously consider them as believable or achieveable. Winners can tell you where they are going, what they plan to do along the way, and who will be sharing the adventure with them."   -Denis Waitley

The Golden Rules For Success 1.Take Responsibility (Who I am, where I am and what I am is totally up to me.) **2.Change** (It is impossible to obtain different results without a change in me and my actions.) **3.Have Goals** (I must determine exactly what I want, how much of it I want and when I want it.) **4.Take Action** (Only my actions will produce results.) **5.Ask** (If I want more from life, I must ask more from life.) **6. Be Smarter** (In order to have more I must do more, and in order to do more be more.) **7.Be Positive** (A positive attitude will always produce better results than a negative one. **8.Be Enthusiastic** (I have a passion for what I believe in!) **9.Keep it in the Right Perspective** (What happens to me does not matter. What I do about it does.)   -Author Unknown

November 26, 2004

Dear Peggy,

Welcome home! I was glad you called last night telling me of your safe arrival home. I'm anxious to get your letter sharing the details of your cruise. Here's an update I said I'd mail on the McDonald's month of November.

I'm still paying the price for my day "quickie" trip to Duluth, before you left on your cruise. That was a cold and drizzly day, but a glorious one. Sharen knew that for almost five years I had been hoping for a trip up north. She gave me a great gift, some time back home. I loved seeing the changes you have made in your home. The furniture, appliances and refinished floors are beautiful. We both wished there was more time.

As I'm writing this, I can smell the warm apple cider and apple cake you had ready for us. Considering I didn't call till we left here at 10:00 a.m., left a message, we were impressed that your were ready for us to visit. The sweatshirt that you had made for Breast Cancer Awareness month and the calico bean soup mix was a nice surprise. I'm happy you are once again busy making gifts for others. Your kindness for others is important.

We stopped at Chub Lake before heading home. It was good to see Marylu recovering well after her major surgery this fall. For six weeks she is restricted on what she can do. Tom, always the greatest husband, has been taking good care of her. Marylu and Tom are Sharen's god-parents. My portable nebulizer that you located for me on the internet made all this possible.

On election day I woke up in such great pain that instead of going to the voting booth, I went to the clinic. I had fractured that same rib as I did in August, only this time the break was "out of line" and the pain was intense. This was the first time since I became "voting age" that I didn't vote in a presidential election. November for the most part has been spent in bed with aches, pains, chills and sweats taking all of my energy, like the old time flu.

This month we've had some special "Good Samaritans." Pat has called many times to say she's on her way bringing dinner. This has happened often this year when I've been sick. Gloria, our backyard neighbor for twenty-nine years, brought over chicken with wild rice soup one night. She didn't know I was in bed with a new infection. She just knew it was a favorite of ours and wanted to share. She also brought over various treats and meals to us this year. (I know you send meals to your neighbor.) What a generous kind gift food is and the staff of life.

Gloria and Larry Carlson are the owners and growers of my "secret garden." Our backyards meet and theirs is always blooming. I am able to enjoy the beauty without the work. Larry had prostrate cancer surgery this summer, and his recovery was slow due to complications. It was a good day when I saw him out mowing the lawn. Good neighbors are a blessing.

November is always a difficult month for me with many memories of special people. As you read your *Guideposts* this month you found a lot of days I had family, as well as baptisms, confirmations, graduation and wedding dates of my kids and grandchildren. Each night when I read my book, when a name and date are listed, I think about that person, their life and include them in that night's prayers by thanking God that our lives have been connected here on earth.

Thinking about all those dates, reminds me that while you were cruising, I called your Jim several times to check on him and what you e-mailed. In one of our conversations he told me that, "He was getting old." I told him, "You better take better care of your health if you want to stay young." I think as long as you are healthy, with only minor ups and downs, or have a disease that can be cured or eliminated you are not aged. The number on the birthday cake only starts to "really" count with chronic disabling or terminal illness. I had various health problems through the years, but not until 1998 at age 70, did I start to feel old. This aging for me started as my ability to fully participate lessened. A good example of this is a friend I have from my lung rehab. Cleo is 91, legally blind, and so full of life. One time in talking to her the subject of death came up. I explained I had no stress about it, I was trying my best, but I was ready to go whenever the time came. She told me, "Not me! I've still got a lot of living to do."

Yesterday, Thanksgiving, was a very special day for us. Nancy and Steve always have this annual dinner for both sets of parents and siblings. She loves cooking a big turkey and all the fixings. We always bring something for the meal. I think some of the pressure is off of the cook by doing it this way.

Steve's parents picked us up for the drive to Zimmerman. Jeff and Shannon no longer can, with two car seats in the back of their car. When we arrived I spotted Sharen's car. It was a great surprise, she and her kids, had driven up that morning and she was busy helping in the kitchen. It was very special having all six grandchildren together for the first time. Counting the twins we were fifteen, five families joined together, Max and Sam's first Thanksgiving. The dinner was the best.

I am glad all my kids like cooking and sharing. They all have made meals for us during the year when I had troubles. I was worried whether I'd be up to going, as I have been in bed most of this month. But by Tuesday things started to improve, I got some strength and we all had a great time. The next day, I ended up with the same troubles, and made a doctor's appointment for Monday. I'm getting concerned how I will be able to pull Christmas together for the family if this continues. I've lost seven pounds in twenty-two days. Just think what it would have been without my Good Samaritans.

Now that you have had your fun in the sun, a break from cancer, I hope you get back to your support group. People with similar problems can gain strength from each other. Keep up the good spirits and positive thinking. Remember, Peggy, you are still young, don't let this disease become a chronic problem in your life. I want you to take care of your health, conquer your disease. There are many more years in your future, this is my nightly prayer for you.

Love always,

Aunt Karen

According to the American Cancer Society, there will be 211,240 new invasive breast cancer cases in the United States in 2005. (40,410 women will die from this disease) There will be 1,690 new cases of breast cancer in men in 2005 in the United States. (460 men will die from this disease) Breast Cancer is the second leading cause of deaths in the United States among women. One woman will die of breast cancer every 13 minutes in the United States. There are more than two million breast cancer survivors in the United States.

In Minnesota, according to the American Cancer Society, 3,200 women will get breast cancer. (700 will die from this disease in Minnesota) In our state, 1 out of every 3 cancers in women will be breast cancer. (48% will be in women over 65 years of age or older; 31% will be in ages 50-64 years of age; and 21% will be in the ages of 49 or younger.)

What is your risk factor of getting this disease? The American Cancer Society tells us that "currently a woman living in the United States has a 13.4% or a 1 in 7 lifetime risk of developing invasive breast cancer. However, a larger portion of the overall lifetime risk is due to the risks at older ages." Eighty percent of all breast cancer occurs in women ages 50 and older. It you are Caucasian, live in North America, are female, then you are at highest risk. African American women have a 1 in 10 lifetime chance of developing breast cancer and have higher fatality rates from not seeking treatment early enough. Ashkenazi Jews have a 1 in 40 chance of developing breast cancer. Asians, Hispanics, and Native Americans have a lower incident rate. Hispanics have a lower incident rate than Asians. Native Americans have a higher fatality rate from not seeking treatment early enough.

"Man's Flight Through Life is Sustained by His Knowledge." -Author Unknown

"As he thinketh in his heart, so is he." -Proverbs 23:7

"Goodness is the only investment that never fails." -Thoreau

"There are people who make things happen, those who watch what happens, and those who wonder what happened." -Author Unknown

"What lies behind us and what lies before us are small compared to what lies within us." -Ralph Waldo Emerson

"We make a living by what we get, but we make a life by what we give." -Winston Churchill

"Ask and it will be given to you; seek and you will find; knock and the door will be opened to you. For everyone who seeks receives; he who seeks finds; and to him who knocks, the door will be opened." -Matthew 7:7-8

11/30/04

Dear Auntie,

Good Morning, Good Afternoon or Good Evening, whatever the case may be. I am writing to tell you in detail about a few more new momentous items we didn't get to discussing on the phone.

On November 8th I saw Seidelmann for a follow up appointment. Did I ever tell you, he called me that night after surgery to check on me? What a dentist! Remember I had a tooth pulled due to a split tooth. It could have been from grinding my teeth when I was sleeping, a poor bite, or maybe a flash of radiation. Anyhow, he's one of the twenty people going to Honduras in February from our former church, Lutheran Church of Good Shepherd. I think it is amazing that all these people from that congregation are giving of themselves. Lois, from radiation, told us they are bringing these diapers made from T-shirts because babies only get two diapers at the hospital. Jim and I donated 30 of our T-shirts for the sewing project Lois is involved with. She also told us that the Honduras people have no electricity or running water. Dr.

Seidelmann is going there to pull bad teeth. There are so many people with needs everywhere this world, Auntie.

I saw Dr. Frye, my young doctor so full of knowledge about radiation oncology, on the 11th, which was my last follow up appointment. We had an interesting talk about my progress, and I tried hard to not to lead him on any medical "bird walks." (I love to do this!) My two areas of skin that got so bad with dry desquamation are much better because of the Silverdene. I called the nurses several times who helped me to get through this issue. Dr. Frye told me that I could come back as needed, but that I should go back to Dr. Krook, my oncologist. He told me the last time I met with him that I could fill my Armidex, my hormone blocker, and I did. I told him, " I haven't had any problems with Armidex and think it's great. I still have hot flashes." I asked him, " Do you want me to stay on vitamin E two times a day?" He answered, "Yes" and we discussed my continuing care with these areas. It was hard to leave Dr. Frye because I knew I may never see him again, and I'd miss his fruitful wealth of knowledge.

That night Jim and I went to the United Way fund raiser with Lisa. The food was lovingly divine. They had wine tasting stations and a silent auction. It was better organized than last year but they didn't have the pasta station and the free gift to take home. This is a great fund raiser for our community.

Another flashback in my mind. On the 12th Jim said goodbye to me as I left on Northwest at 7:00 a.m. It was hard to leave Jim at home, as I knew he'd miss our daily adventures dragging me all over like his personal rag doll.

Back at our cedar brown house, Jim on Saturday had the Woodland Hills Cougar group rake our yard. They had done garden work this summer for us and did an excellent job. Jim had to get up early to remove the landmines from the yard. In the spring they are coming to do some more garden work.

Jim was so lonely that he e-mailed me many times a day. He is a true blue "people person." I tried to write him and my computer friends, as often as I could on the ship.

Jim kept busy going out with friends and family. He ate some of the many hot dishes I had made ahead for him. Jim even worked at the Christmas City of the North parade for the Duluth Police department. He kept busy with his many activities including fixing his truck that broke down.

On my arrival home from my trip, Jim, my adult children and puppies were very welcoming. Jim had a note on my bed from the puppies and pink flowers for me. The trip was wonderful but as we all know, "there's no place like home." While flying home on Thanksgiving, I thought of how much I have to be grateful for (stable health, family, friends, and experienced doctors). I missed Thanksgiving dinner arriving home too late. My only consolation was the first class meals on the plane. My new luggage was lost but found the next day in Minneapolis.

Another exciting appointment with Dr. Krook, my oncologist, on the 30th. He was his usual humorous self as he checked me over and we talked extensively. I will be going back in March for a mammogram and extensive blood testing. He's such a funny, cool doctor. It was Dr. Frye who told me, "They don't make doctors out of the same mold as him anymore." He is right. Did I ever tell you that Dr. Krook sends letters to his patients in the mail after a visit? I think this is a nice personal touch. Remember one school I worked in where the teachers had to call the parents the first week of school to introduce themselves and state positive comments? This was also an attempt to work with the parents before a crisis occurred.

Oh, I had an appointment with Dr. Bloom, my gynecologist. He's such a sweet, kind doctor. I've seen him a few times as I have some concerns about my bladder getting worse due to lack of hormones. I brought him a book to show him about hormone balance, a well debated issue. Auntie, I sure miss those hormone pills!

The Citizen's Patrol party is at Lakeview Castle Tuesday and I'm looking forward to it. I want to eat some real Greek food.

Next year I'm going to plant a tree or shrub in my garden that the Cougars are going to dig. I will finish my poem, even though I'm not a well seasoned poet since college.

"I know the road back

Because I know the road there

This is a true story of

A breast cancer survivor

Finding her way

By the people who lived

Through it deeply."

There's a lot of light at the end of my tunnel, and I feel I have learned so much. I've learned to cherish each precious moment, value the people I care about, to continue to set goals for myself that are not stressful, to be more thoughtful toward those who have made a difference in my life, to make a difference in other people's lives, and to understand the path that all human beings have walked.

Love,

Peggy

December 20, 2004

Dear Peggy,

As I am writing this, I'm listening to the CD you sent me from your trip, "Cruising Collection, Caribbean Nights." Another Monday without rehab, but the doctor said to wait until Jan. 15th. I hope the rib is healed by then, my muscles are disappearing fast.

I'm glad that we agreed last year to stop exchanging gifts and use the money for charity. This year I increased my Christmas Salvation Army check that I mail to avoid the kettles. But I have also started to do as Nancy always has, donate to each kettle she encounters when shopping. Our grocery store has one, so I "hit the green" often.

Last year I sent a check to Mt Olive's Sunday School. It's my way of showing appreciation for the years our children, as well as myself as a child, were in their Christmas programs. The school director's reply impressed me, so I sent another check this year. The children had been raising funds to send a horse to a family in Kazhikstan and a calf to a family in Africa.

Our family has a long history with Mt. Olive. In 1921 your Grandpa Prahl sold his hardware store in Brownton to move to Duluth, to be a Marshall Wells salesman. After Mom and Dad built their home in Hunter's Park, sometime before 1930, he transferred his Missouri Synod membership to Mt. Olive, and stayed a member until his death in 1953. We continued as members of Mt. Olive until we moved down here in 1974.

Mom and Dad had a great art of compromising. They were both Lutherans, but from different synods. Mom's synod at the time was "The Norwegian Lutheran Church of America." Mom wanted to stay a member of the church as she had so many ties to Zion Lutheran from childhood. One Sunday, Mom would pick me up after Sunday School and we would go to her Zion church services. The next Sunday Dad would meet me after Sunday School and we'd stay for Mt. Olive's services.

Another example of their compromising was their voting. Dad always voted Republican, Mom usually Democratic. Many times they would cancel out each other's vote. Neither of them had a problem with it, each respected their spouse's opinion. Compromise is such an important part of a happy and contented life.

This writing about happiness and contentment brings me back to why our family made changes in our gift giving several years ago. It had gotten to be stressful, I felt all the shopping, deciding what you had to buy each person, making sure each received equal dollar amounts, plus all the wrapping had become too time consuming. This activity left little time for the real "Present" of Christmas.

Now at Thanksgiving, each adult puts their name in a bowl with three suggestions on it. Whoever draws your name, doesn't have to use your ideas, if they choose not to. Nancy, our "shopper-shopper," had a difficult time with this. She still wanted to give each family member a gift. We compromised by instead of Grandma filling everyone's stockings, I'd just do the grandchildren. Each adult would bring a stuffer for the other adult stockings. We all still gift to the children under 18.

Jim and I started to give checks to Sharen and Nancy to buy their children's gifts from us. But we didn't play the game well, we still kept shopping for the big kids and spouses. I kept Max and Sam on our list as I wanted do our own shopping for their first Christmas. This year when the Grand Rios Indoor Water Park opened here in Brooklyn Park, we made reservations for four poolside rooms. That took care of all that shopping for the big ones. A big plus, their restaurant would be open in time for Christmas dinner and brunch on Sunday. No cooking of a big dinner by me. This sounded easier last fall, before my November " knock-down."

It was mid December before we headed out with our Christmas shopping list. We found the umbrellas and leather gloves we had decided to buy as our stocking stuffers and got a few things. Jim's not interested in shopping except at the grocery store. Later, while I was on the phone with Ellie, I found we had only one men's extra large glove, Steve's size. My good friend quickly offered to pick me up with the glove up to make an exchange. After we exchanged the gloves, we worked on my list. Ellie even carried in all the packages because of my rib.

On Saturday, I decided to wrap the shopping that was still in bags, stuffed in my closet. Unbelievable, but in wrapping Steve's gloves I found under the band two right hand gloves. Jim wanted to know, "How two women could be so stupid?" I told him, "No dumber than you and I, buying one glove." That night Ellie and I headed out for a third time for one pair of gloves. The sizes and colors were all mixed up, so we ended up on the floor on our hands and knees checking the bottom racks. On the way home she took me on a tour of many homes decorated for Christmas.

My "Good Samaritan of the Month" Ellie, got me to my perm appointment when our car unexpectedly ended up in the shop. We had numerous trips to get the gifts and I still needed stocking stuffers for each of the grandchildren. Ellie, a breast cancer survivor for 13 years, retired early this year. Our friendship goes back twenty years when we both worked at Brooklyn Park City Hall. She is a friend I can always count on. I would never have managed this Christmas without her help.

Later that day Gloria, our back yard neighbor, brought over six kinds of homemade Christmas cookies. A dozen of each to share with our family at the resort. Her angel cut outs are almost too pretty to eat. We were ready for the holidays because of friends help and kindness. Time for two special affairs, to enjoy Christmas programs on TV, and most of all, time to spend with the "real reason of the season."

This week is the annual Lung Power Christmas luncheon at Unity Hospital. An opportunity to meet others in rehab at different times. Terri's last day as a case manager for lung rehab will be on the 29th. She has been one of my case mangers for over five years. Pam and Terri made such a great team. They have helped so many lung patients by their knowledge, concern, and encouragement. Terri is a breast cancer survivor of three years. She will be missed by many.

Thursday night we are going to Linda and Gary Bahr's annual Christmas get together. They were our next door neighbors from the day we moved in. Several years ago they moved to a new home, but they continue this get together. Along with the Carlson's, Linda's Mom, Gerry will be up from Florida for the holiday.

182

Yesterday I made the list of what we need to bring this weekend. All the meds and equipment remind me why we don't travel. Ellie and I will share Christmas Eve church services. We have always spent Christmas Eve together since the kids got married and spend that night with their spouse's families. Christmas day, after the Laphams arrive, we'll load up the car and check the resort to see if our rooms are ready.

I hope the Andersons have a great Christmas and Santa is good to all. But Peggy, don't overdo it. Recovery from three surgeries takes time. Write when you have time on how your holidays went.

Love,

Aunt Karen

"When things get rough remember--it's the rubbing that brings out the shine."
-Author Unknown

"The primary cause of unhappiness in the world today is...lack of faith."   -Carl Jung

"Nothing will benefit human health and increase chances of survival of life on earth as much as the evolution to a vegetarian diet."   -Albert Einstein

"If you haven't any charity in your heart, you have the worst kind of heart trouble."
-Bob Hope

"When you cease to make a contribution, you begin to die."   -Eleanor Roosevelt

"Kind words can be short and easy to speak, but their echoes are truly endless."
-Mother Teresa

"Constant kindness can accomplish much. As the sun makes ice melt, kindness causes misunderstanding, mistrust, and hostility to evaporate."   -Albert Schweitzer

12/31/04

Dear Auntie,

Happy New Year or should I say it in 12 hours, as it will be the year 2005? So much has happened this year. I'm not going to dwell on cancer in this letter. Instead I'm going to talk about the joys of life. It was good to hear from you the other night. How was your Christmas at the water park resort? I'm anxious to hear all about it. It's so important to cherish family and friends as they give us the proper perspective and appreciation of life.

You made me feel better the other night when I was frustrated about not losing weight. Your comment, " You're developing muscles and toning your body first," made me feel a lot better. I walk three miles a day and see little progress with my weight. One hour of exercise a day is really important, but I read that a person needs to walk 10,000 steps for it to make a difference. I want to lose weight to improve mycancer prognosis.

December has been a busy month. The Citizen's Patrol Christmas party at the

Lakeview Castle went great. Bible Study is very interesting. We have walked almost halfway for the Duluth Clinic Heart walking program. Maybe we will earn a T-shirt yet. This next week I have Miller Dwan Breast Cancer Support group, and I will meet with Kim Storm from the YWCA Breast Awareness Program. Jim found someone else to answer phones for the WDSE fundraiser, so I didn't have to answer phones after all. I've been busy writing letters, buying and making Christmas gifts, knitting and trying to eat better. On the 14th of December we had another potluck at church with several groups. It was fun because we made gift bags with cookies and fruit for shut-ins for Christmas. Our church really cares about their members. Later on that day I went to see my family physician, Dr. Nisswandt.

I read an interesting article in the *New Yorker* magazine on Dec. 13, 2004 titled, "The Picture Problem." It tells the reader that the radiologist looks at cancer for two different patterns, "They look for lumps and bumps, and they look for calcium." When cancer grows it produces calcium deposits. Radiologists look at all types of calcium deposits. The article goes on to tell that it's the irregular calcium that is laid down inside a tube that is cancerous. Cancer cells are ragged. Another article was about a study done by the *University of Washington Harborview Medical Center* of ten board-certified radiologists. They had to look at 150 tissue samples of 27 women with breast cancer and 123 with healthy breast tissue. The differences in diagnosing was amazing. The article tells the reader that radiologists need more rigorous training and experience. The problem lies with mammograms and the reading of the x-ray. There are gray areas, and we as patients need to understand this.

Life keeps me busy. Helen and I went on the 15th to a luncheon at the Radisson with our retired Central Group. On the 16th I had physical therapy with Lois due to the lymphedema in my arm. This was from shaving a single hair under my arm, flying or radiation. Who knows? Jim had Police Reserves and bell ringing at the mall that night, so I had fun shopping until I dropped. His group is thinking of having musical instruments to play next year, so they can collect more money for the Salvation Army. Two more potlucks on the 18th and 19th. Jim on Tuesday had the HAM X-mas party at STC. Jim, I, Ray, and his new wife, a UMD professor, took care of the food. Then on the 22nd Jim had his school class party. Jim, I and Ken (a retired plumber), got the party all set up. Ken and his wife gave us a beautiful box of homemade cookies as they did last year. I do miss making cookies and candy but I keep telling myself, **"No, sugar fuels cancer!"** Thank goodness we went to the Scandinavian weekend up the shore to buy a few cookies. Jim had an appointment in the afternoon in regards to his physical, so I went with him. I had PT again on the 23rd. Then on the 24th, we went to the Pickwick for an early free patron appreciation buffet that started at 11:00 a.m. Life is good!

We celebrated Christmas Eve at our house and delayed Christmas Day until Sunday as Chris had to work. On Christmas Eve, I made beer basted prime rib with horseradish sauce. Joel and Lisa made popovers and I made a spinach salad as I was thinking anticancer foods. Also I had made sour cream chive mashed potatoes, and carrots in ginger sauce because I know ginger is an anticancer food. The appetizers were olives, olive mix or fruit in phyllo cups, crackers with garlic, garlic dip and spinach herb dip. The beverages included lemon water (Lake Superior Cocktails), Godiva (white chocolate liqueur), and wine that Lisa and Joel brought. We got Rosa Regale (BANFI) made with raspberries and rose hips because it's my favorite and has antioxidants in it. I made a new recipe of lemon bars with mint leaves on top that Chris wouldn't keep his hands off of them. Mint is another anticancer food also!

Chris made home made gifts and labeled them with things like "To the lucky receiver, from the humble giver…God Bless us, Everyone!" I'm wondering if he was thinking of the time he was Tiny Tim in the Duluth Playhouse.

The next day was Christmas Day and I surprised Jim with a loaf of Twig Bakery bread in his stocking. That's what he wanted Santa to bring him. You know, we don't exchange Christmas gifts, instead we give money away to our favorite charities. I wish my family would get more into stocking stuffers instead of gifts. I fill their stockings, but they don't fill mine. Jim and I spent the day at home thinking of a trip for next Christmas.

Sunday, we called it Christmas Day, Lisa, Joel, Chris, and Betsy came over. (Lisa and Joel had their traditional goose dinner on Thanksgiving, and Jim missed not having a turkey dinner.) I ordered a free range turkey from Old World Meat Market where I get unradiated hamburger. The menu included a stuffed turkey with traditional stuffing and corn pudding like Jim's mom use to make. We had the old layered ribbon jello salad, fresh garlic buttered broccoli, asparagus hot dish, rosemary turnips, a fresh fruit salad for antioxidants, leftover wines, coffee, cookies, and candy. Broccoli and rosemary are anticancer foods as well. You see why I enjoy traveling on the holidays?

The following week on the 29th was another potluck at church. It seems like I'm always eating. Tina, from Younkers, did my hair for the New Years Eve party at the DECC, and did I look young! We are going to dinner at Porters Restaurant with three other couples first.

My friend, Donna, had surgery recently, and she sure has gone through a lot with her type of breast cancer. She's in a lot of pain and it's enough to bring you to your knees to pray. You wonder "Why her?" I found talking to her was important. It was important for me to reach out to her and have a heart to heart conversation with another woman. I think it's important to share your fears and give each other support.

I read an article on breast pain management from *Cancer Treatment Centers of America*. It told the reader that chronic pain can last for three months due to the nervous system, anxiety, depression, and insomnia. It didn't mention the cutting of tissue, muscles, and nerves, which surely must be the reason. A study from the University of Wisconsin on pain called me a few times in the fall. I do think shooting chronic breast pain lasts longer.

Hope everything is going well with you. Write or call when you can. I'm going back to being my own creative, intuitive person. I am no longer a short term task person, but I stay with it, focusing until I get to the meat of the project. At times I catch myself tuning out, and I have to get back on that merry-go-round ride of life.

I'm still going to physical therapy because I have lymphedema.

God Bless.

Love,

Peggy

Here's some lymphedema information. (Isn't this what Aunt Clara had?)

Cancer Facts, Terms, Knowledge, and Concepts

Symptoms:

Lymphedema-A chronic condition of abnormal swelling of the arm or leg due to the disruption in the normal lymphatic flow or circulation. It occurs from build up of fluid and thick protein in the tissues that forms like sludge or garbage. It causes you be at risk for infections and slows the healing in your body. It can occur at birth, after surgery, after an accident, or after radiation. If it gets past stage one, it is permanent.

Lymphedema Symptoms: Swelling in the arm or leg results in restricted mobility, tightness of clothing or jewelry, numbness, heaviness, feeling of pins and needles, pain, and resulting anxiety or depression. Call your doctor if you get a red, hot or swollen arm immediately!

Primary Causes-Unknown causes and at birth.

Secondary causes-Infection, trauma, following surgery or radiation.

Serious Conditions from Lymphedema: Heaviness, deformity, repeated infections, cellulitis and lymphangitis.

Removal of Lymph Nodes-You can get blockages and scar tissue because the nodes filter the lymph fluid.

Diagnostic Procedures/Treatment:

Complex decongestive therapy (CDT)-This is when you use lymphatic drainage and compression garmets.

Exercises of Lymphedema: The American Cancer Society recommends the following three exercises after breast surgery after consulting your doctor, a physical therapist or occupational therapist.

1.Hand Walk-Stand facing a wall 6 inches from the wall. You take your ten fingers and have them walk up and down the wall. Do this several times.

2.Shoulder Flex Exercise-You lie on the floor and reach 180 degrees above your head. You may have to work your way up to this.

3.Floor Arm Exercise-You lie on the floor on your back with your arms parallel and down to your sides. Keep your arms straight, raise them over your head, try to touch the floor above your head at 180 degrees. You may have to work your way up to this. Do several repetitions.

Four Things to Not Do After You Have Your Lymph Nodes Removed:

1.Never let anyone take blood pressure from the affected arm.

2.Never allow anyone to draw blood from this arm.

3.Never allow anyone to put an intravenous line (IV) into this arm.

4.Never allow anyone to give you a shot in this arm.

Treatment of Lymphedema:

1.Manual lymphatic massage draining

2.Compression bandaging

3.Compression sleeves (custom made or the simple sleeve)

Lymphedema Treatment-Avoid lifting more than ten pounds, never use a hand razor, treat all cuts with antibiotics immediately (carry antibiotics and bandages with you), never have blood tests, shots, IV's and blood pressure taken on this extremity, wear gloves when working in the garden or in the house, use DEET spray to prevent bites and stings, use a thimble for sewing, be careful with knives, nails, scissors, screwdrivers, and saws, wear a compression sleeve when traveling, be careful with household chemicals, avoid stove burns, keep your hands free of possible injuries, don't go in a hot tub or pool (only with caution), don't wear tight things around your wrist or arm, use tanning lotion or avoid excessive sun, wear a compression sleeve to reduce swelling from working, exercising, and flying.

Medical Findings/Terminology:

Cellulitis-This is a severe bacterial infection caused by staph or strep that can occur from lymphedema. (Women have died from severe cases of this!)

Function of the Lymph Nodes-The function of the lymph nodes is to remove harmful bacteria and germs, produce white blood cells that combat bacterial and viral infections including lymphocytes.

Lymph-A protein rich fluid.

Lymphadenitis-Inflammation of the lymph node or this area.

Lymphanhgitis-A bacterial infection of the lymphatic channels that can occur from cellulitis.

Lymphatic System-The system involved with the lymph, lymphatic vessels, and lymph nodes throughout your body. It carries circulating lymph fluid to fight infections and fights immunity toward diseases.

Lymphatic Vessels-These are vessels found primarily in the neck, armpit, groin, front of elbow, and behind the knee that remove the excessive fluid and proteins from the spaces between the bodies cells. The vessels return the fluid back to the blood's circulatory system after being filtered.

Lymphedma-A serious problem that can result from axillary lymph node dissections. Only 10-25% of the women who have axillary node dissection develop it. It's rare with a sentinel biopsy.

Lymph-edema-Lymph is the natural body fluid and edema stands for swelling.

Primary Lymphedema-This type of lymphedema occurs at birth, adolescence or later in life.

Prognosis-Prediction for the outcome of the disease and chance of recovery.

Secondary Lymphedema-Occurs after cancer surgery or radiation.

Lymphedema

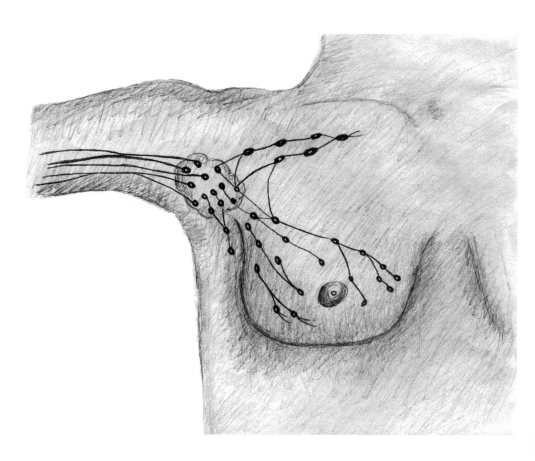

Lymph Drainage Can Be Blocked By Scarred Ducts
And A Build Up Of Lymph Fluid

Lymphatic System

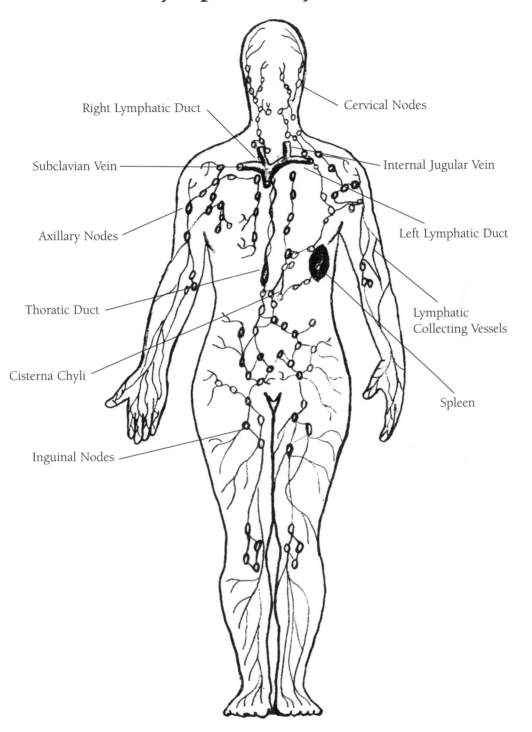

Cervical Nodes

Right Lymphatic Duct

Subclavian Vein

Internal Jugular Vein

Axillary Nodes

Left Lymphatic Duct

Thoratic Duct

Lymphatic
Collecting Vessels

Cisterna Chyli

Spleen

Inguinal Nodes

Lymphedema or secondary lymphedema can occur from the removal of lymph nodes in breast cancer. Lymph drainage becomes disrupted and the nodes cannot be regenerated. The body does try to find ways to compensate for this loss. The tissues are deprived of the nutrients that they need and cannot get rid of the waste products. Lymphedema may not occur after surgery or radiation. It can occur years later. There are different stages of lympedema. They include: **Stage 0 which is the latent stage.** There is no edema at this stage. **Stage 1 is mild and a reversible stage.** There is swelling from the protein like fluid that has build up in the arm, back, or chest wall. A patient or doctor can put a dent in the skin from this stage. It will not stay at this stage if the patient does lymph drainage exercises. **Stage II is an irreversible stage.** The swelling is in the tissue, fibrosis has begun and sclerosis has developed. Indentations in the skin no longer disappear. The tissue has become hardened and permanent. **Stage III is called severe lymphedema or elephantiasis by some sources.** The swelling is extreme, there's inflammation, and the skin is hard or fibrotic, has growths, bulges, and does not heal. You can get cellulitis and die from it. Septic is a life threatening infection you can get and the symptoms can include: blotchy coloring on the skin, redness, a very warm feeling, and pain.

There are **grades of lymphedema**: 1.pitting edema 2.pitting edema 3.pitting edema 4.pitting edema.

Who Get Lymphedema?

Between 12-35% of all breast cancer patients will develop lymphedema. Some sources state the percents are lower. If you have 20 or more nodes removed you are at risk for lymphedema.

Treatment of Lymphedema:

There are several ways to treat lymphedema. They include: 1.compression garments as a sleeve or gloves 2.mechanical pumps 3.manual lymph drainage using a light touch approach 4.elevation 5.medication 6.diuretics 7.antibiotics 8.Steroids 9.benzopyrones 10.liposuction 11.surgery 12.laser surgery 13.experimental treatments 14.bandaging.

Lymphedema Precautions:

1.Never have your blood pressure, blood tests, IV's placed in this arm, or shots taken from this arm. 2.Always keep your nails clipped. 3.Avoid sharp tools and animal scratches. 4.Use bug spray. 5.Do not over strain these muscles and never lift more than 20 pounds. 6.Wear gloves when gardening or working outside. 6.Wear your compression sleeve when flying, exercising, or doing tasks that would agitate it. 7.Do not go in the sauna or hot tub. 8.Don't lay out in the sun, use tanning beds, and do use sunscreen. 9.Be careful with various types of massages. 10.Do not wear tight jewelry around your wrist or arm. 11.Eat a healthy diet, low in salt, high fiber, don't drink or smoke, eat plenty of fruits and vegetables. 12.Maintain a normal weight. 13.Avoid stressful sporting activities. 14.Measure your arm for changes. 15.Wear a sports bra. 16.Keep this arm clean. 17.Don't overstress this arm.

January 1, 2005

Dear Peggy,

Happy New Year! It's 2005 and we're still alive. I hope you and Jim had fun celebrating New Year's Eve. You have much to celebrate this year.

Today Jeff brought over the twins for a visit. Shannon stayed home to paint a Mural on the nursery wall. The boys are both sitting up. Max, while on his back, digs his heels in and can scoot around. Sam's not interested in that game yet. They are such happy babies and so full of smiles.

I haven't been able to spend as much time with the boys as I would like. My frequent lung infections, fracturing my rib twice this fall, and fungal problems has made me more careful before the twins develop more immunity. Fungus is not contagious, but I worry that some of the lung infections could be.

Jim must have had too much fun with all the Christmas cookies and goodies for a diabetic. He ended up at Urgent Care at our clinic. It was only after many tests did we learn his blood glucose had spiked to 535 early in the morning.

Peggy, I know you are getting anxious to lose weight but good nutrition, your walking the mall plus other exercising will bring results. Actually, what is lost over a longer period of time is better for your health and easier to keep off as these better choices will become a habit of your daily life.

I know you will keep up with your follow up appointments, mammograms and whatever else is needed to keep on top of this disease. But, remember this, if cancer does reoccur you are a fighter and you will overcome. Don't forget, I've been counted out a few times these past few years and I'm still here. Don't ever get discouraged or give up, you are needed and loved by many. Take care.

Love always,

Aunt Karen

Everyday we look at the back of cans and packages to see more chemicals that we don't have the slightest idea what they have in them. Our bodies seem like chemical holding tanks for these ingredients. Supposedly, they are regulated by the FDA, but then we read on the news that this drug or that drug has been taken off of the market. We can control what we eat. **A diet high in natural grains, fresh fruits, vegetables, low fat dairy, organic, natural, or low fat protein sources is the best.** We as consumers need to ask ourselves, "Are these the choices that our ancestors would of eaten? Are we eating a bunch of chemicals?"

Cleaning supplies were a lot different years ago. I remember when common household products such as vinegar were used. Today our cupboards are filled with a wide variety of chemicals to clean every imaginable item in our kitchens and homes. The old ways were better. **We need to go back to natural cleaning supplies. In the kichen we should....**

1.**Get rid of aluminum cookware** as traces of it can get into food, and aluminium can have an effect on an individual's mental cognition.

2.Plastics as plastic wrap, plastic bags, and containers leach into food when heated. They contain polyvinyl chloride (PVC), polyethylene (PE), polyvinylidene chloride (PVDC) and plasticizer. Cover foods in the microwave with paper toweling that has not been recycled. Cool all food before freezing it and placing it in a plastic bag. Don't defrost meat on PS-polystyrene foam meat trays as they leach. Never use plastic containers with a 3,6 or 7 at the bottom. Do not use number 7 pitchers or containers. **Limit or eliminate plastic and use safer alternatives as glass containers.**

3.Bleaches, chlorinated scouring powders, dish soaps, drain cleaners, and other cleaners contain petrochemicals in them. **Instead we should use biodegradable, water based, free of phosphates, and free of propellant cleaning products.**

4.Water is chlorinated and has floride in it. The National Cancer Institute has said that florinated water can produce cancers, and a medical college in Wisconsin has stated that some kinds of cancer have contributed to chlorinated water. Tap water can contain a variety of things it it as bacteria, heavy metals including lead, atrazine (a hormone disruptor), radioactive particles, radon, chemical residues, organic chemicals, chlorine bi products, industrialized wastes, synethetic arsenic, and even gasoline solvents. **We are far better off drinking filtered water or safe choices of bottled spring water.**

5.It's so important to wash all food-fruits, vegetables, and I've even seen that one should wash meat. Rembember some fruits and vegetables have pesticides on them. Organic choices do not use pesticides.

January 16, 2005

Dear Peggy,

Your busy month of December sounded great, but I hope you are not forgetting to take time to "smell the roses." A priority for you must be taking time to relax and not always going at life with full steam ahead.

No matter how much we plan ahead and organize, things can change in a hurry. Christmas Eve morning brought the news that Max and Sam had croup and weren't able to join us for their first Christmas. Shannon went to her family's dinner that night, leaving Jeff in charge. They reversed roles that next night, so Jeff could join us for dinner on Christmas and deliver their gifts.

Linda surprised us later with a decorated Christmas roll wreath. She has done this many years, but at their party they gifted us with a container of homemade snack mix to share with the family at the Rios. Good neighbors and good friends have really blessed our aging and ailing lives.

After Christmas Eve church services, Ellie and I usually pick Jim up and have dinner at a Chinese restaurant. This year I surprised her by having dinner ready here. Other years when having all the family for Christmas dinner, the tables would already be set. I had made a salad earlier and put a frozen lasagna in the oven before we left for church. The oven heat and steam from things boiling on the stove can cause breathing problems for me, but I'd be gone when it's baking. This was the first time ever that I didn't have a tree. I missed putting all my special ornaments up, some going back to when I was a child. I had some decorations up and we played my Christmas tapes during dinner.

The kids, big and little, loved the Rios, Minnesota's largest indoor water park. There's something for all ages as the "Lazy River" to float on, waterfalls to play in, and many exciting slides. A "Hurricane" serpentine tube slide, at up to 45 MPH, zoomed you down three stories before dropping you into a funnel bowl and ending in a pool. This was a challenge not all of us took.

We arrived at the hotel early after being told when we called, "Come on over." We were astounded with the mass of humanity. The lobby was jammed. The long, very slow, hardly moving lines of people waiting to check in was endless. The line kept growing as we kept waiting.

My early reservations for dinner, (first made in their book for that date), and reconfirmed the day before, ended up in another big wait. The hostess said she would join two tables together to seat six and the other four at a nearby booth. I explained this was my family's Christmas dinner. I had been assured we would be seated together for their family style dinner, served on platters, and that this was not acceptable. She rudely replied, "I can't accommodate you." I said, "We'll wait." There were a lot of empty tables and booths. In the row she wanted to seat six of us, at the third table a couple had just started to read their menus. I thought she could handle it. My "no cooking for me" dinner was going down hill fast. We waited and waited until the girls finally had to ask for the manager, when the hostess told them, "It's not my problem." A booth table was quickly pulled over to join the other two tables to make seating for ten. The next night we ordered in pizza by the pool with all the "goodies" we had brought. I find it hard to understand how some people are always willing to go an extra step to keep an agreement, while others can't be bothered.

The gifts were great, everyone had neat ideas for the stocking stuffers. It seems by giving less, more thought is put into the gifts. For the first time in three years, I didn't end up with pneumonia after the holidays.

The story behind my favorite Bible verse goes back to 1939 when my Sunday School teacher was Dr. Pohl, who had recently immigrated from Germany. At Christmas he gave each of his class a wine colored fuzzy cardboard plaque. In our class of seven students we each received a different Bible verse written in white letters. Mine hung on my bedroom wall for many years. It became a part of my nightly prayers, and I think about it in stressful times. **"....His name shall be called Wonderful, Counselor, Almighty God, Everlasting Father, Prince of Peace."** --Isaiah 9: 6. This verse reminds me in my own words, that gets changed from time to time, depending on my thoughts, that God is …

Wonderful - God's wonder is awesome, starting with the miracle of each birth.

Counselor - Who we go to first for comfort and strength.

Almighty God - There is no higher or greater power.

Everlasting Father - Always forgiving, always there for us.

Prince of Peace - Only through God can we have peace of mind, body and soul.

I hope Duluth is as lucky as we are. So far we have had only ten inches of snow and never more than two inches at a time. Our neighbor, John Thomson, who kept us plowed out for so many years is recovering from a heart attack. Keep warm, slow down, keep all those appointments.

Love always,

Aunt Karen

The Highest to The Lowest Incident of Breast Cancer
Diagnosis By Race

According to American Cancer-Per 100,000 women from 1997-2001 statistics

High
Caucasian 141.7
African American 119.9
Asian Americans and Pacific Islanders 96.8
Latinos 89.2
Native American 54.2
Lowest

A Woman's Risk of Developing Breast Cancer

American Cancer   2005 Probability
Lifetime Risk--We have a 1 in 7 lifetime risk of developing invasive breast cancer.
60-79 years of age--1 in 13 chance of developing breast cancer.
40-59 years of age--1 in 24 chance of developing breast cancer.
Birth-39 years of age--1 in 20 chance of developing breast cancer.

Breast Cancer Deaths

According to The American Cancer Society, "The chance that breast cancer will be responsible for a woman's death is 1 in 33 (3%) . In 2005, about 40, 410 women and 460 men will die from breast cancer in the United States. Death rates from breast cancer have been declining." There is a 1 in 13 chance 13%) of getting breast cancer if you are over 60 years of age.

"A cheerful heart is good medicine, but a crushed spirit dries up the bones."
-Proverbs 17:22

"He who is plenteously provided from within, needs but little from without."
-Johann Wolfgang von Goethe

"Has any man attained inner harmony by pondering the experience of others? Not since the world began! He must pass through the fire." -Norman Douglas

"The purpose of life is not to be happy--but to matter, to be productive, to be useful, to have made a difference that you lived at all." -Leo Rosten

"We are what we repeatedly do. Excellence, then, is not an act, but a habit." -Aristotle

"Nothing can bring you peace but yourself." -Ralph Waldo Emerson

"You may have to fight a battle more than once to win." -Margaret Thatcher

"Let food be your medicine, and medicine be your food."
-Hippocrates, "Father of Medicine"

1/31/05

Dear Auntie,

I'm wondering how that flamboyant little Brooke is doing in the hospital. Is she off oxygen yet? How is her pneumonia? To be six years old with asthma and pneumonia is pretty scary. Pneumonia can surely suck the energy out of an adult let alone a child. I hope she is doing better. Nancy and Steve must be very worried, as Zack must be about his little sister. Do you think her going to all of Zack's hockey games in the cold arenas could contribute to her pneumonia? You know, we with asthma have to be very careful breathing cold air into our lungs. That's why it's so important to dress warmly and cover our mouths with a neck scarf.

I've been filling out my relicensure forms to renew my teaching license. I took at least thirty credits in 2003. Some were semester classes and are worth more than quarter credits. I cried all the way to the board of education to turn in my forms. Teaching was a big part of my life but it involved a lot of stress.

Have you heard from Sharen? How are Emily and Landon doing? I'm thinking about Landon cooking the squirrel in the crock pot, and I'm wondering if he has tried any of the recipes in the *A Man Can* cookbook I gave him. Also, I've been thinking about Emily and her friend managing the wrestling team. I wonder if the boys on the team know she has a black belt in karate.

I'm a little tired today as I woke up at 5:30 a.m. with the crows squawking, and they sure are early morning pickers. Lisa and Joel are in Minneapolis, so we had to go and let her Corgi dogs, Chester and Chloee out. They are staying at a ritzy hotel called Le Meridian. They even have a plasma TV and telephone in the bathroom with down blankets on the beds. Lisa and Joel went to the play, "The Miser," at the De La June Luene theater, in which Lisa's friend, Sarah had a part. I guess Lisa is taking students to a play there this spring. Also, Lisa and Joel went to Sister Fun, ate at Cosmos and the French Meadow Bakery. Sounds like they had a good time.

I got an e-mail from Jim's sister, Kay and she wrote to George Solomon, the Las Vegas singer who sat on her lap several times during a show on the cruise. He wrote, "Thank you Kay for the kind words and the comfortable lap! Love, George." He was a ball of fire and could really sing!

Faith sure is a pact with the Almighty. Faith Lutheran has opened their loving hearts and arms to me, and I want to love them back. We were ushers at church yesterday and we signed up for a few more times. Next we walked the mall for the Duluth Clinic Heart Walking program, went on errands and did some grocery shopping. Today we are going to the Center for Personal Fitness, and I have my writing class. Jim and Gerard Scofield meet for their "weekly business meeting."

On Saturday Jim and I went to Wendy Braun's father's funeral, Terry Ruse. It was at the Cremation Society of Minnesota. I was really impressed with the packed room and so many people that it over flowed into two more rooms. Family members and friends stood up and told true stories of Terry. My friend, Wendy, told of her dad having his four girls play football with the boys across the street. Terry told his girls, "Be strong." I'm thinking that's what we all have to be in this life. Another story came from a nephew who dropped spaghetti off the cook stove at the cabin onto the dirt floor. Terry told him, " Pick it up and stir it." As everyone was eating it, he then winked at him and said, "A little dirt never hurt anyone." I can picture in my mind this happening. It made me think there is a lot of dirt along the way, and we just need to forget about it.

We went to Junior Achievement on Thursday night to a wine tasting party with two other couples, the Lassilas and Arndts. They had great appetizers, there were items to bid on and even non-alcoholic wine do drink. Everyone seemed like cannibals eating and drinking their prey. We hope next year we can get two more couples to go, so we can get a sit down table and two bottles of wine. It was a lot of fun, and it's great to have a network of friends who care about people, life, and our community.

Friday night was the Police Reserve Party at Black Woods in Proctor. I brought home five T-shirts from the different events. The Duluth Police Chief was there, as well as the assistant, and Herb Bergson, our Mayor. The Mayor thanked the Police Reservists for the activities they had participated in. We sat with the same people as last year, Doc Hogan and his wife, and Mr. and Mrs. Ethier.

Our church on Saturday night had another pot luck. We brought chili that Jim had made and watched the movie, "The Boys Next Store." It was rather interesting.

I called *Life Extension* on the 25th as I was concerned about my triglycerides which are the high fat levels found in a person's blood. I wanted to know if high triglycerides could contribute to hormones in your blood, as I read balanced lipids effect your hormone balance. I know that estrogen goes in the blood and into the fat tissues. *Life Extension* told me balanced hormone levels are important. Also, I wanted to find out if testing for estrogen, progesterone and testosterone were standard tests during physicals. These levels tell if women need to go on hormone replacement therapy (HRT). I had read somewhere when women become estrogen dominant, the progesterone drops, and that's when breast cancer cells can develop. (More women are estrogen-progesterone positive in breast cancer diagnosis.) Maybe as women, we need to have this checked. *Life Extension* will test your blood by sending it to a lab if you are a member. I've also read that insulin and estrogen together create a strong effect in your body. It's important to lower your glucose and insulin to decrease the estrogen effects. Back to my triglycerides, after finding a *Life Extension* article on triglycerides, I decided to take fish oil each day. Oh, I even asked them the question about excessive testosterone in men and prostrate cancer. The answer was "Yes." Men should have these levels checked!

I'm still trying to lose weight by walking three miles everyday, and some days it's very hard. Who would think that obesity and a sedentary life style can contribute to breast cancer? I don't want my prognosis to be poor, so I'm going to lose weight. When I got breast cancer my weight was 189 pounds and now I'm down to 173 pounds.

After talking to *Life Extension,* I decided to see Dr. Nisswandt, to discuss having my blood tested for triglycerides and see if they do test for hormone balances. I wanted to see her about my constipation from prescriptions, gastric reflux burning problems, and my lymphedema under my arm and in my upper back area. I am wondering how to control inflammation which I see as a problem. (Recently I feel like I have constipation of the brain!) Problems, problems, concerns, concerns.

I also read some information about triglycerides in *Remedy* magazine. Triglycerides are found in your body tissues and blood stream. When triglycerides are high they stop the leptin messages from going to the appetite control center. That's why it's hard to lose weight when you are leptin resistant. I also read in Ellen Moyers book, *Cholesterol and Triglycerides,* that lipids are effected by estrogen. Studies have shown that when we take estrogen, triglycerides rise. Some researchers feel that it makes it harder to remove cholesterol because estrogen alters the HDL as well. Isn't this interesting?

Diet, the most common word in households today. I am now controlling my diet by eating more fish than ever, very little red meat, lots of fruits and more vegetables than ever. I'm forcing myself to eat more grains, but it's hard. I drink purified water, skim milk, green tea, vegetable and fruit juices, and I drink this green algae called Green Goodness that I buy at Cubs. It's full of 14 phytonutrients. There's spinach, green tea, broccoli, apple juice, pineapple juice, mango, banana, kiwi, lime juice, Jerusalem artichokes, garlic, lemon, algae, and various grasses in it, to name just a few ingredients. I'm thinking about a fact I read, which said forty percent of all cancer victims die due of malnutrition. That's a lot!

I did make a doctor's appointment for next week. My calendar is getting filled up again. Monday night I have my writing class with Rhonda, my teacher, who is so full of energy, and we'll be doing critiques. Tuesday is my Breast Cancer Support group through the Duluth Clinic at Miller Dwan, and I'm looking forward to it. This Saturday we are going out to dinner and the play, *Blithe Spirit*. We will be going with a group of seven couples. Jim and I haven't seen a play in a real long time.

Recently on the internet, I found where you could send for free lymphedema bracelets. I sent for the braclets, and I talked to Lois, my physical therapist, about them after showing her the letter I drafted. Then I dropped the lymphedema admittance bracelets off with a letter stating the importance of lymphedema bracelets being put on patients when they are admitted to the St. Mary's hospital. Hopefully they will use them. I feel more lymphedema education is important in our community.

Oh, you'll laugh at this one. Lisa went to an appointment with Dr. Nisswandt, and they were talking about the breast cancer T-shirts or sweatshirts I made. Lisa told her she encouraged me to, "Wait till next year and do a better T-shirt." She then told Dr. Nisswandt I said, **"No, I'm not doing T-shirts next year as I'm going to be over breast cancer!"** I was thinking it was easy to put this all behind me.

I read the findings on two studies in a report from *Life Extension* that compared ultrasound, mammography versus MRI in detecting breast cancer. The first study involved 192 women and detecting cancer. The mammography and ultrasound detected 6 out of 9 cases of cancer, whereas MRI detected all 9 cases. The MRI is

204

far better according to the Kuhl et al. 2000 study. Another study involved 196 women at high risk for hereditary breast cancer and compared them with three types of diagnostic equipment. The mammography detected 2 out of 6 cases, the ultrasound detected 3 out of 6, and the MRI detected all 6 cases in the Warner et al. 2001 study. Interesting.

Lots of blue skies, green lights, warm days, and times to sleep in the streets....as a radio show would once say.

I'm enclosing a copy of my new breast cancer diet and food pyramid that I made up from many sources. We should both try to eat these natural foods. It's a good plan for me, but may not be for some breast cancer survivors or cancer patients. I think you'll like the vitamin and mineral chart that I came up with. Hopefully you are receiving these nutrients in your diet from natural sources, or you may need to supplement your diet with pills. Please look carefully at it.

Love,

Peggy

*-Indicates strong anti cancer foods
**-Indicates foods eaten by our maker or from our ancestral diet

Fruits-(6-8 servings per day)
Apples***
Apricots,**Avocadoes
Bananas, Berries
Blackberries
Blueberries*
Cantaloupe*
Cherries
Cranberries*
Dates*
Figs**
Grapes-purple-*red-*green-**black
Grapefruit, red *
Honeydew
Kiwi
Lemons*
Melons**
Nectarines
Oranges*
Plantains
Peaches*
Pears
Plums
Pomegranates*
Prunes
Raisins
Raspberries*
Strawberries
Watermelon*

***Beans-(2-3 x's per week)**
Adzuki, Azuki beans
Black eyed peas
Black bean spread
Black, white beans
Chick peas
Dried/ Fresh tofu
Garbanzo beans
Great Northern beans
Lentils-green-brown-red
Lima beans
Minestrone soup
Mung beans
Navy beans
Peas (dried)-Soup
Pinto beans
Soybeans**
Spirulina
Tofu
Tempeh burgers
Vegetarian burgers

Dairy- (1-2x's a day)
Skim milk **
Low fat yogurt **
Butter-raw or ghee

Beverages-after each meal and between
Black tea,* Arizona Green tea, white tea
Green tea-**(3 x's a day)
No caffeine, grain coffees only
Pomegranate juice, V-8 juices
Purified water, Naked juices
Seltzer water, Bolthouse Green Goodness

Supplements-daily
Multivitamin*
Indole 3 tablets*
Green tea tablets
Vitamin E*

Protein-(3-4 x's per week)
Bass
Cod*, calamari
Eggs
Fish**
Flounder
Haddock*
Halibut
Herring
Mackerel*
Organic Liver
Orange Roughy
Perch
Poultry-free range/hormone free

Red meat-(3 oz.)/grain fed/hormone free
Salmon*
Sardines*
Snapper
Sole
Tuna*
Trout

Pasta
Condiments/Herbs/Other**
Basil*
Bee pollen-in moderation **

**Grains/Whole/Cracked/Ground/
Rolled)-(2-3 x's per day)**

Amaranth
Barley **
Bran
Brown rice
Buckwheat/bulgar
Chapatis
Corn grits
Crackers
Cracked wheat
Ezekiel bread

Flat bread
Kamut
Millet
Mochi
Natural cereals
Oat groats
Oat meal*

Polenta
Popcorn
Rice*

Cinnamon, cardamom
Curry, cumin, chili pepper
Flax seeds*
Fish oil
Garlic**
Ginger*
Horseradish*
Hemp
Kelp
Lecithin (licorice)*
Mint*
Mustard*
Olives**
Olive oil* , oregano
Parsley*
Primrose
Rosemary*
Sage*
Sesame, soy
Spearmint
Turmeric,* vinegar

Rice cakes
Rolled oats
Rye/flakes
Quinoa
Spelt Wheat
Teff
Tortillas
Wheat**
Wheat germ*
Wheat kamot
Whole oats
Wild rice

Vegetables-(4-5 servings per day-organic)

Acorn squash
Alfalfa*, argula
Asphagus
Artichokes
Arame
Argula
Asparagus
Beans, green*
Beets*
Bittercrest
Bok Choy*
Broccoli*
Broccoli rabi

Potatoes*
Pumpkins*
Rutabaga
Radishes- red*
Onion
Red clover*
Romaine lettuce
Rutabagas
Salsify
Scallions
Sea cress
Sea palm
Shepherd's Purse

208

Brussels sprouts*
Butter head lettuce
Cabbage-*red
Carrots*
Cauliflower*
Celery
Celery root
Chinese broccoli
Collard greens
Corn*
Cucumber
Daika greens
Dandelion greens
Dulse
Eggplant*
Endive
Escarole
Fennel*
Ferns
Green beans
Green leafy lettuce
Kale*
Kelp
Kohlrabi
Leeks
Mustard Green
Mushrooms-shittake
Nori
Onions-red**
Ocean ribbon
Parsnips, green peas,*peppers*

Snap peas
Spinach*
Sprouts,* soy*
Squash-various *
Sweet potatoes*
Swede
Swiss chard
Tomatoes *
Turnips
Turnip greens
Wakame
Watercress
Wax beans
Yam
Zucchini

Nuts**
Almonds
Chestnuts
Hazelnuts
Nut butters
Pecans
Peanuts*
Pine nuts
Pumpkin seeds
Seed butters
Sesame seeds
Sunflower seeds
Walnuts*

My Food Pyramid

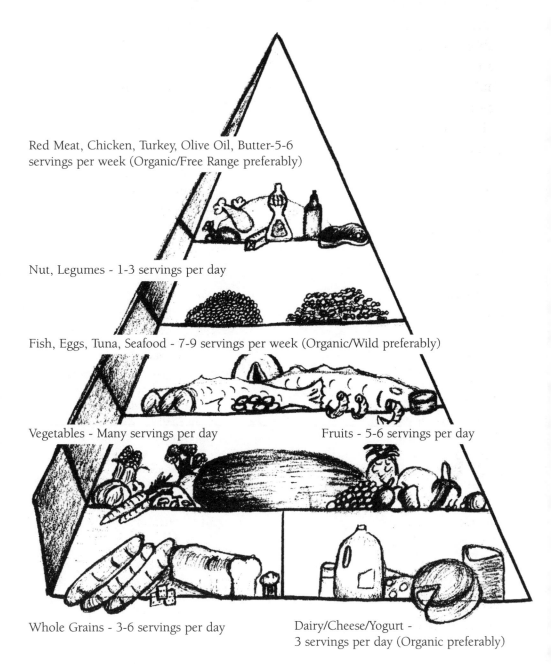

Red Meat, Chicken, Turkey, Olive Oil, Butter-5-6 servings per week (Organic/Free Range preferably)

Nut, Legumes - 1-3 servings per day

Fish, Eggs, Tuna, Seafood - 7-9 servings per week (Organic/Wild preferably)

Vegetables - Many servings per day

Fruits - 5-6 servings per day

Whole Grains - 3-6 servings per day

Dairy/Cheese/Yogurt - 3 servings per day (Organic preferably)

Supplements - under the direction of your doctor
Beverages - 8 glasses of water a day, caffeine free green and black tea, V-8 juice, Boathouse and Naked drinks, tomato juice

Alpha Linolenic Acid-Sources: flaxseeds, flaxseed oil, pumpkin oil, soy and walnuts. These are thought to reduce inflammation, and they may protect you against breast cancer, and protect your immunity. It is thought by French researchers that breast cancer patients who have a high content of alpha linolenic acid in their breast tissues are less likely to develop metastases.

Beta-Carotene-Sources: green or yellow fruits and vegetables. Beta-Carotene is thought to reduce the risk of breast cancer. Research studies have shown that a low intake of arytenoids may be associated with increase risk of breast cancer. Research has also shown that women's risk of dying can be decreased if they have a high intake of beta carotene.

Capsaicin-Sources: chili peppers. This is thought to stop tumor promotion in lab tests. It can reduce inflammation, increase healing, is antibacterial, can be used as a pain killer, and is an antioxidant.

Flavonols, Polyphenols, Catechin, Theogallin, EGCG-Sources: beans, berries, black tea, and green tea. A major medical school found no association between Flavonols. These are thought by many sources to be anti-tumor promoters, to help with cellular enzyme activity, and cause reduction in nitrosamine formation.

Geinstein-Sources: legumes, soybeans. Some call them soy isoflavones. These are thought to reduce the risk of hormone positive cancers and stops angiogenesis. The Chinese have done studies on these, and they work. Supposedly, geinstein has a anti-estrogen effect by binding estrogen receptors. It's considered a weak estrogen agonist. (Ask your doctor first, if you are estrogen positive until more research is done.)

Indoles-Sources: broccoli, brussel sprouts, cabbage, cauliflower, horseradish, kale, kohlrabi, mustard greens, rutabaga, spinach, turnips, and watercress. These cruciferous vegetables are thought to reduce hormone positive breast tumors by stopping or inactivating the estrogen with their anticancer properties. They also increases glutathione-S-transferase activity, stop the growth of certain cells possibly because of 13 c. These foods contain sulforaphane, are rich in nitrogen compounds, and are a good source of other nutrients as well.

Isothliocyantes, Sulforaphane-Sources: boy choy, broccoli, brussel sprouts, cabbage cauliflower, Chinese cabbage, collards, kale, kohlrabi, mustard greens and radishes, rutabaga. These are thought to stimulate enzymes that convert estrogen to a benign form, they block steroid hormones, and stop the production of breast cancer.

Organosulfur Compounds, Allelic Acid-Sources: cruciferous vegetables, garlic, leeks, onions, and watercress. These are thought to reduce breast cancer, induce certain enzymes, and inhibit tumors production.

Phenolic acid (Ellagic Acid)-Sources: berries, celery, citrus, cruciferous vegetables, eggplant, flaxseed, fruits, grains, licorice root, nuts, parsley, peppers, soy, tomatoes, and whole grain. These are thought to prevent cancer and limit tumor formation from studies on animals.

Quercetin-Sources: apple skins, bell pepper, grape juice kohlrabi, onion, pear skins, tomato leaves, and wine. Quercetin and other flavonoids have shown to reduce breast cancer as well as be an antioxidant. They also can increase bone density in women. Considered a phytoestrogen it attaches to estrogen receptors but doesn't stimulate them. Other flavonoids like naringenin and nesperiden are thought to inhibit breast cancer as well. They are even thought to help prostrate cancer.

Vitamins:

Vitamin A-5000 IU-**Sources:** broccoli, carrots, green leafy vegetables, fortified milk, and liver

Vitamin B (Thiamine)-0.8 mg.-1.5-**Sources:** dried beans, enriched grains, whole grains, pork, and sunflower seeds

Vitamin B2 (Riboflavin)-1.1-1.7 mg-**Sources:** enriched noodles, liver, milk, mushrooms, and spinach

Vitamin B3 (Niacin)-14-20 mg-**Sources:** beef, bran, chicken, enriched grains, mushrooms, peanuts, and tuna

Vitamin B5 (Pantothenic Acid)-2.5-10mg-**Sources**: animal tissues, cereals, legumes, and whole grains

Vitamin B6 (Pyridoxine)-6mcg-15 mg-**Sources:** animal proteins, bananas, broccoli, and spinach

Vitamin B12 (Cyanocobalmin)-2-6mcg-**Sources:** animal products

Vitamin D -400 IU-**Sources**: catfish, egg yolk, halibut, herring, mackerel, milk (cow milk, canned, and soy), oysters, pudding, salmon, sardines, shrimp, shitake mushrooms, sun exposure, tofu (enriched), tuna, and yogurt

Vitamin C-30-160 mg-**Sources:** broccoli, cantaloupe, citrus fruits (oranges, grapefruit, lemons, and limes), green peppers (raw), potatoes, strawberries, and tomatoes

Vitamin E-30 IU-**Sources:** butter, brown rice, corn, cottonseed oil, corn oil, nuts, soybeans, soybean oil, vegetable oil, and wheat germ

Vitamin K-0.03 mcg/kg-**Sources:** green leafy vegetables, liver, and is also made by intestinal bacteria

Cyanocobalmin-2-6 mcg-**Sources**: animal products

Biotin-60-300 mcg-**Sources:** cauliflower, cheese, egg yolk, and peanut butter

Folic Acid-160-300 mcg-**Sources:** asparagus, avocados, bananas, beans, beets, brewer's yeast, brussel sprouts, cabbage, calf liver, cantaloupe, citrus fruits and juices, Endive, fortified grain products, garbanzo beans, green leafy vegetables, lentils, sprouts, and wheat germ.

B Complex-varies-only take if not taking vitamin C, Thiamin (B1), Riboflavin (B2), Niacin, B6, and B5 (Pantothenic Acid)-Sources: various, see above

Choline-425 mg-**Sources:** breast milk, cabbage, calf liver, cauliflower, egg yolk, garbanzo beans (or chick peas), kale, lentils, oatmeal, peanuts, soybeans, soy lecithin, and wheat germ.

Inositol(Myoinositol)-_____-**Sources:** breast milk, calf liver, cantaloupe, citrus fruits, dried beans, garbanzo beans, lentils, milk, nuts, oats, pork, rice, veal, wheat germ, and whole grain products.

M (B9)-400 mcg-_____

Minerals: (Needed for cellular metabolism, growth and healthy body.)

Calcium-700-1200 mg-**Sources:** broccoli, dairy products, dark green leafy vegetables, legumes, milk, sardines, and turnip greens

Phosphorous-800-1200 mg-**Sources:** cheese, dairy products, grains, lentils, meats, meat products, milk, nuts, poultry or chicken breasts, processed foods, and soft drinks,

Potassium-(200 mg)-**Sources:** bananas, broccoli, green beans, oranges, orange juice, peanuts, meats, milk, mushrooms, several fruits, and sunflower seeds

Sodium (Salt)-2,400 mg-**Sources:** bacon, beef, bread, butter, canned foods, clams, green beans, ham, margarine, milk, olives, pickles, processed meats, salted nuts, sardines, table salt, and tomatoes.

Magnesium-200-400 mg-**Sources:** beef, broccoli, cashews, green leafy vegetables, kidney, legumes (dried beans and peas), nuts, popcorn, spinach, tofu, wheat bran, and whole grains

Iron-8-18 mg-**Sources:** eggs, enriched bread, lean meats, liver, legumes, green leafy vegetables, kidney beans, raisins, and whole grains

Zinc-12-15 mg-**Sources:** beef, cereals (bran flakes, oatmeal, raisin bran, and rye), cheese beans, chicken, beef, crab, eggs, lamb, lobster, milk, nuts (cashews, peanuts, pecans, pumpkin seeds, sesame seeds, sunflower seeds), oysters, and pork

Chromium-.05-0.25 mcg-**Sources:** fats, meats, peanuts, oils, oysters, shrimp, turkey, whole grains, and vegetables

Copper-2-3 mg- **Sources:** cereal, drinking water, filberts, lamb, legumes, liver, meats, pecans, peanuts, pork, oysters, foods, seafood, seeds, and walnuts

Selenium-0.05-0.2-**Sources:** grains, kidney, liver, meats, sea foods, and seeds

Manganese-2-5 mg-**Sources:** cereal products, fruits, green leafy vegetables, legumes (dried beans), milk, nuts, seafood, seeds, tea, vegetables, whole grains, and yogurt

Molybdenum-0.15-0.3 mg-**Sources:** beans, breads, cereals, milk, and in other foods

Silicon (Silica)-29-30mg-**Sources:** apples, barley, beets, beans, bell peppers, brown rice, cucumbers, fruits (skins), green leafy vegetables, leeks, legumes, nuts, oats, onions, parsnips, root vegetables, seeds, and whole grains.

Iodine-150 mcg.-**Source:** iodized salt

*B6 and niacin can be toxic if you have too high of doses. A, D, E, and K are stored in your lipids and too much can lead to toxicity. Fat soluble vitamins act like hormones. High doses of vitamin E can produce high levels of artery clogging LDL cholesterol and lead to an increase in LDL and triglycerides.

February 10, 2005

Dear Peggy,

Brooke is back in school but her continuing problems are a concern. The thought of a six year on a nebulizer is very upsetting. I keep reading how asthma can be controlled but she struggles. Maybe I should mail the book you sent when she was in the hospital as I haven't seen them lately.

The book you sent me, *The Will and The Way*, covering forty years of changes in Duluth, published by Manley Goldfine and Don Larson is great. Reading about Duluth is always a pleasure to me. As a secretary to Bob Morris at the Chamber of Commerce, I remember doing preliminary work for the future Port Terminal. This was my first job after college. I found it exciting to be involved in so many of Duluth's activities. The Goldfine family has certainly been a leader in supporting and improving our home town. I remember when Dad would call Erwin and Manley the "boys" when their dad's store one of his sales accounts.

On the phone you asked why I called my anti-fungal meds my "designer drugs." That's because of the price. The last time I picked up my prescription for Voriconazole it was $2,118.49 for sixty pills, a one month's supply. I do take many prescription medicines, most in the "race to breathe." This is the seventh month I have been on it. I'm finally getting some strength, breathing better, keeping my voice, the limb pain and other symptoms are clearing up. The fungus is not gone, but with my meds and by pacing myself I'm able to do more.

Thanks to our government recognizing the services of retired veterans, we have an excellent prescription plan with a low co-payment. We only see the price of the drugs we buy locally. The long term ones we order through the mail. My best estimate for my ten prescriptions and Jim's diabetes and heart meds are over $3,000.00 a month. Without good prescription plans, some people can't afford to take their needed medications. Many seniors have only Medicare, and I can't see how that will be much help when you have high priced drug needs to survive. "The golden years" can get tarnished pretty fast with high costs of prescriptions. It also concerns me the problem with some employers not offering health benefits. The insurance is very costly, unless you get group rates. The young people just starting out on their own have less income, in many cases, and can't afford insurance.

I think it is a shame that our drug companies claim they need high profits for research when they spend hundreds of millions of dollars advertising drugs on TV and in magazines. We can't buy these advertised drugs without a doctor's prescription. Let's give our doctors some credit to know what drugs we need based on their experience.

This morning when I paid the bills, I decided to increase my annual gift to the National Jewish Medical and Research Center. This organization is a leader in respiratory illness and in children's asthma. In their last newsletter, I read about their breast cancer research and thinking of you I made a change.

I'm not very generous or interested in supporting groups with a high percentage of operating costs. Unfortunately, too many groups spend a large share of our donations for high salaries and promotional material that keeps filling our mailboxes. Many times little of what we give is actually used for research or to help others.

Those telemarketers soliciting on the phone are a big pain. I now request any caller to send me a copy showing what percentage of donations are used for their operating cost before I sent a check. So far, I haven't received any responses. Peggy, I know you and Jim have always supported many charitable groups, but I think we all should be "picky" on what we do.

I am thrilled that you are writing this book with no compensation to fight breast cancer. Your time and expenses are well spent for such a good cause. I have some concerns about my letters being included in your book. I hope my thoughts don't offend anyone. But as you know, I write from my heart, just as it is to me. Happy Valentine's Day to all the Anderson's. Hope you have a great day.

Love always,

Aunt Karen

P.S.

My pen pal, Lillian, sent me two tapes of her singing hymns. She even included my favorite, "Holy, Holy, Lord God Almighty." A great gift sharing your talent with others. She is a hospice volunteer in Texas and a former classmate.

Ways To __Increase__ Breast Cancer Risk

1. Drink 2-5 alcohol drinks per day and very little water.
2. Lead a sedentary life style with very little exercise. (This way you can't excrete estrogen and toxins from your body.)
3. Continue to be overweight by eating a high fat diet of saturated, unhealthy and processed foods. (This way your body can't fight the enemy.)
4. Continue to choose a contraceptive that makes some women at risk. (This depends on the type of contraceptive, age you went on it, and your hormonal level.)
5. Don't pay attention to high dose HRT that increases some women's chances of getting breast cancer. (It will depend on if you have too much estrogen in your body from HRT, and possibly from phytoestrogens and environmental estrogens.)
6. Continue to use certain cosmetics, hair dyes, face creams, shampoo, and deodorants that have been linked to cancer.
7. Work and live in places that are under study for breast cancer.
8. Continue to make poor life style choices. (Examples include chemical laden drinking water; breathing air from tobacco, factories, and vehicles; using unhealthy cleaning products; using herbicides and pesticides)
9. Continue to live a stressful life that runs down your immune system.

Ways To __Decrease__ Your Chances of Breast Cancer--That You Have Control Of

1. Have mammograms, clinical breast exams, do breast self exams (This should be three days after your menstrual cycle or the first of each month if you are post menopausal.), and ask your doctor do hormone monitoring.
2. Eat a plant based diet rich in darker fruits (at least 6) and a variety of colorful vegetables (at least 5) per day. Eat at least 35 grams of fiber per day, as fiber binds the estrogen as it goes through your intestines. Avoid highly laden estrogen and growth hormones in meat, poultry, and dairy sources by eating organic or low fat choices. (Your daily fat sources should be 10% or less to reduce the estrogen level in your body.) Eat all the necessary natural nutrients you can in your diet and supplement if necessary. Drink clean filtered and purified water to help your cellular structure.
3. Look at what can cause you to have breast cancer before it happens. (ie-If you have dense breasts, if you've had atypical hyperplasia, or lobular carcinoma in situ.)
4. Don't drink or smoke.
5. Exercise at least 4-5 hours per week and have a very active life style. (Exercise stimulates the immune system, reduces stress levels, and reduces estrogen levels in estrogen based breast cancers.)
6. Don't let yourself get overweight, in case you get breast cancer.
7. Work on your breathing, so your cells have a lot of oxygen. (Thanks Sally!)
8. Avoid unnecessary toxins in your life and environment.
10. Know ahead of time your family cancer and breast cancer history.
11. Be aware of your age, gender, and race factors for getting breast cancer.

"The best and most beautiful things in the world cannot be seen or touched--but are
felt in the heart."   -Helen Keller

"The Best Things in Life Are Free
    When we count our many blessings,
    it isn't hard
    to see
    that life's
    most valued
    treasures are
    treasures
    that are free.

For it isn't what we own or buy that signifies our wealth. It's the special gifts that
have no price: our family, our friends, and health."   -Unknown Author

"Love Conquers All Things."   -Virgil

"Your vision will become clear only when you can look into your own heart."
                                                              -Carl Jung
"Love bears all things, believes all things, hopes all things, endures all things, Love
never ends,"   -Unknown Author

"My grace is sufficient for you, for my power is made perfect in weakness."
                                                      -Corinthians 12: 8-9

"To keep a lamp burning, we have to keep putting oil in it."   -Mother Teresa

2/15/05

Dear Auntie,

    Belated Valentine's Day! When you are going back to see your U doctor? I hope

you are going to talk to her about building up your immunity to fight the fungus. We

really need more nutritional doctors to support our regular family physicians, so they

can help us. It seems the family physician needs to know a lot about everything, and

I'm sure this is hard.

    We have a lot of toxins in our food, water, and air. Air quality is important to our

homes and environment. It's important to avoid people who smoke as there are risks

with second handsmoke. The clinic has a spot for smokers to smoke, but it makes me mad to have to walk past smokers at the hospital and clinic. At the hospital recently some man blew his smoke in my face as I tried to avoid him. I don't go out when the pollution level is high, since I have asthma, and I avoid breathing in extremely cold air unless necessary by covering my mouth. We sure have less pollution in Duluth than Int'l Falls with the paper mill and Athens, Greece with their car emissions.

A little nutrition 101 for us. Toxins in water are a concern to me as well. I know fish can pick up mercury, so we need to be careful with the fish and fish oil pills that we eat. (It's one reason I don't buy farm raised salmon.) Some big companies are still contaminating our waters by dumping sludge into them, and others are burning dioxins that go back into the water through the atmosphere. Filtered water is important, and my water purifier is now a part of my kitchen sink. At some point, Jim and I are going to have our water tested. We have been drinking quality bottled water for a long time due to the lead pipes in our older home.

Food contamination is a concern according to the American Cancer Society. Foods can also have toxins on them from pesticide sprays. When I bring home my fresh fruits and vegetables, I wash them right away before putting them away. (Jim doesn't even wash his grapes!) We love eating more fruits and vegetables than ever before. Dietary habits are so important for cancer prevention. Jim eats a lot more grains than I do! Poor nutrition and alcohol weakens the bodies defense mechanisms. Coffee, which we love, dehydrates the bodies cells. I've read many articles on foods, pesticides and toxins, and the jury is still out on some of this research.

Protein is a whole new subject. Growth hormones (with estrogen) are injected into animals to fatten them up, so that they have heavier poundage of meat to sell at the market. We have limited our amount of beef and poultry to a low fat diet, and I try to buy free range chicken, buffalo (low in fat), and un-radiated beef (from Old World Meats). American Cancer states in their literature that people should eat a low fat diet with a limited amount of red meat, but preferably eat a vegetarian diet. I have read in nutrition books that New York strip, top sirloin and T-bone are better cuts of meat with less fat in them. We should always try to eat organic meat. If we do buy meat, we should buy low fat cuts of meat and the leanest hamburger we can buy. Pork is not a big part of our diet anymore. Instead, I eat a lot of safe seafood choices. We all need a certain amount of protein but we shouldn't be eating excessive amounts.

As for dairy products, I've cut down on all dairy products that once were a big part of my diet. I now choose low fat dairy. Dairy products can also have toxins and growth hormones in them as well. Remember that animals eat grains, and they can have pesticides and toxins in their food from the spraying. We don't eat very many processed or packaged foods anymore.

The *World Health Organization* has stated that cancer can be from poor nutrition. My diet has improved as I have gone from not eating saturated potato chips, fried foods, fast foods, burnt food, licorice candy, pop, and cookies to eating healthy natural foods. I see mothers as I once did coupon shopping for cheap junk foods to feed their families. My immune system needs to fight and destroy those bad boy free radicals. Years ago our ancestors were gathers of fruits, vegetables, nuts, and hunters of fish, and they ate a limited amount of meat. We all need more fresh fruits and vegetables, unprocessed high quality foods in our diet, a smaller portion of low fat meat, whole grain choices, vitamin supplements and more fish in our diets. I read that breast cancer patients are often low in vitamin A, low in wholesome grains, and their foods are too high in fat. I think sugar is killing America because it's raising the blood glucose levels of Americans. As a society we are obese, have more diabetes than ever, and sugar is fueling breast cancer. All this can be prevented.

On the internet I read recently about a population study that found dietary factors increase one's risk for cancer. They included animal products, meat, total fat, saturated fat, dairy, refined sugar, total calories and alcohol. In reading this article, the following factors lowered your risk for cancer: fish, olive oil, whole grains, soy, legumes, cabbage, vegetables, nuts and fruits. I know when I eat anything with sugar and don't walk, my hot flashes get worse. Maybe we should all eat a Mediterranean diet. Our diets effect our health.

In my refrigerator I keep a bowl of fresh frozen fruit from Sam's Club. I add drained bottled fruit, fresh cut fruit, and canned fruit to give it added flavor. On my cruise I ate a lot of fruit, and now Jim is eating more because it's right there in the refrigerator. Fruits are really important for detoxification and fighting the free radicals in a persons body. As far as vegetables, I keep a bowl of fresh cut vegetables in the refrigerator to eat freely. I'm trying to eat more colorful fruits and healthy vegetables rich in antioxidants and phytochemicals. The deeper the colors the better and richer the value. I hope you are eating enough low sugar fruits and vegetables.

The American Cancer society feels overweight women should lose weight by exercising and eating a strong plant based diet. I need to lose weight, so that my fat cells are not full of elevated hormones that cause an imbalance in my system. My Armidex is helping to fight this cancer war in my body.

Drinking water, breathing, and getting sunshine are important for a cancer patient. I'm forcing myself to drink more water each day to flush my system out. Sometimes I drink cold lemon, lime or orange water from the refrigerator. It's a way I can trick my mind into thinking, I'm drinking something healthy and elegant. I need to work on my breathing exercises and take a meditation class. I do pray, if that counts.

The Monday night before last, I had my writing class, and I brought my story "The Trail of the Paper Carrier." I also gave my paper carrier a tip and a copy of the story. He wrote me a thank you note stating he thought it was great. That helped my esteem a little. (Self esteem… I read somewhere women who eat a lot have low self esteem because it makes them feel good.) In class we will be critiquing our stories and then rewriting them. I'll send you a revised copy.

On the first Tuesday night of the month was our Miller Dwan Breast Cancer support group. It was open discussion, and we talked about other ideas for speakers in the future. Some ideas included a radiologist, a pathologist, a nutritionist, a specialist in lymphedema, and a nutrition tasting party. Possibly, there could be an open discussion on why women get breast cancer, with each woman bringing in the reasons on how she thought she got breast cancer. When I got home, I thought of other ideas that would be good as sharing a favorite breast cancer or health book for a book talk. Everyone could bring in something to share with everyone else --like a story, a poem, positive affirmations or thoughts to live by. (The teacher is coming out in me!!!)

Sharon Lassila called the other day, and we discussed the cruise she and Jerry are going on. It seems like everyone is going on a winter trip except us this year. Jim and I decided Ireland will be our next trip as we can fly free with our points and take our whole family. Lassilas have had to go to Ely a lot on weekends as Jerry's dad is ill.

Later this month I have to go back to see my family doctor about a lot of things. She is a doctor that listens to my many concerns, as I may of told you before. I asked her about having my triglycerides retested. My triglycerides are down to 269, so they are still high. My liver enzymes are up, so I have to go in for another blood test in a month. I joke at the registration desk and often state, "I am no longer a professional student but a professional patient." They see me all too often.

This disease has given me a second chance on life by the gift of time. I have been blessed throughout my adult years with a truly rewarding teaching career, the gift of knowing many dedicated professionals in the teaching profession, and knowing many caring adults in the community in which we live. My life experiences have invigorated me to do my best for others. I realize we all have hopes and dreams, and we all want to make a difference in our society. I think what we do for God is our gift back to Him, just like the quote you once sent me, "What we are is God's gift to us, what we become is our gift to God." I have never forgotten another of your quotes, "The crop you sow is the crop you reap." (This is a little revised from the Bible verse.) You told me that your mother often said this quote. I think we are all on trial to do our best in this life. God probably has lessons along the way for us, and I do believe that faith healing is important.

Valentine's day went great. On Sunday eve, Jim said chuckling gleefully, "Honey, you pick out the pink carnations that you adore, as I don't want to get the wrong ones." At sunrise on Monday, I looked up as he handed me a card and said, "You are my rock, my pillar, I love you very much. Then he said, Happy Valentine's Day!" as he then handed me the card. See he does go to the ends of the earth to please me most of the time. It made me feel special.

I recalled the evening before how he secretly bought the card at Walgreens, sneaking it snuggly into his greenish jacket pocket so I wouldn't see it, as we trudged along to his truck. He acted as it was a top shelf secret.

At other times, I can cook up some unsavory words about him. After him cooking all summer, it is now my full time job. I'm glad we have had the same visions and values in life along the way. He somehow thinks it's his mission in life to bring me back from the atomic bomb scars like the Hiroshima Maidens to blessed reality. I have the scars to show, but I have my life experiences that must mean something. This breast cancer situation has rocked Jim's life as well as mine, but I think he's learning to deal with it. His sister Kay bought him the book, *The Breast Cancer Husband* by Marc Silver, and he diligently reads it. At times he asks me questions like, "How do you feel?" At other times he tells me, "I want to be involved every step of the way." Jim wants to be active in my treatment, and I couldn't of asked for a better person on my team.

Smokey Joe and Peanut Butter look so cute in their buzzed off hair cuts. They are walking around the house with their pink scarves with red hearts that I made for them. I have a lot of new ideas of gifts I can make for people when I'm not busy typing and researching. For example, our vet said that there are about twenty dogs a year that get breast cancer (or mammary cancer) from not being spayed. One of our dogs years ago had this happen. These dogs need breast cancer scarves!

Yes, I'm still trying to motivate myself. I have to kick myself to go but I do enjoy walking at the Center for Personal Fitness while listening to *My Grace,* a Thrivent CD and other religious CD's. Cancer really teaches us that life is of value, and we all need a lot of hope and faith. My gentle yoga class starts at 6:30 a.m., and it's helping me with my breathing which is so important to a cancer patient with lymphedema. Jim came home from work and the first thing he asked me was, "Did you go to your "yoge class?"

Gentle yoga class is going great. I hear my instructor's voice, Tamara, telling us in her very powerful words "think the world is beautiful…," and I drift off in my own meditation. After class I decided to tell her that there were some things I couldn't do. I told her because I didn't want her to think I was "a lazy student." I explained about my breast cancer surgery, radiation and lymph edema, as I didn't have strength to do activities on the left side due to weak and tight chest muscles. She held my hand and told me with her sweet voice, "Don't think you can't do it, think of …." I thought what a positive instructor. It's great to see the colorful sunrises looking at the hillside of Duluth as we stretch, breath, mediate, and do our gentle yoga exercises.

I know, I need to do regular exercises from having breast cancer surgery to build up my strength. I do have intermittent daily pain and my underarm burns at times. I'd like to take a Feldenkrais method class to work on my breathing in February, or the arm and back class in March. I asked Jim about taking the Mindfulness Based Stress Reduction class in the spring at the clinic. It's a class for stress, anxiety, and chronic pain. It involves meditation, yoga, stretching, awareness enhancing exercises, along with group activities and assignments. Jim felt I had too much on my plate right now.

I just want to tell you Auntie, that you have been the best aunt, best friend, and my best spiritual advisor in life. You have made an impact on me by touching my life in so many ways and because of you, I am who I am. You have listened to me day after day talk about this relentless enemy, namely cancer, and how to shoot it down, so I can go back forward with my life. Thank you, Auntie!

Cancer is not going to ruin our family. Each of us must deal with it in our own way, and it can be a growing experience. In some cases, it has been very hard on my children, but hopefully they have grown from this experience. We have extraordinary blessings in our lives by our own will, as well as the will of God. I feel I value life, people, and others more. I feel God has given me a second chance. We're having soup suppers at church during Lent, and it's a real educational experience. I also now belong to the church's prayer chain.

Chris was over the other night to pick up his laundry before work. He told me, "I can't take my laundry because it will get cold in the car all night." The complex layers of life. Thanks for praying for me.

Love,

Peggy

February 22, 2005

Dear Peggy,

Your homemade valentine with your special message is a keeper. The thoughts you expressed really touched my heart. My angel is on my jacket, and I can't wait to take a bath with the darling roses. I'm sure you know where I put the special book mark. Thank you for remembering me.

The heart shaped card reminds me of people with "a good heart." By that I mean people with compassion and caring for others. Both you and Jim raised your children showing compassion for others. I often think at Thanksgiving of the time all four of the Andersons were at the DECC serving dinner for the needy. Jim was Santa Claus. Your Jim has done so much with volunteering with Police Reserves and other activities in the community. Peggy, you have always been a ready volunteer, even while teaching full-time, and kept busy making gifts for others, gifts that come from the heart.

I think it was pretty neat that time when you, Jim, and Lisa took on a paper route to lose weight. For every pound you three lost, you donated a pound of butter to the food shelf. They got thirty three pounds and you got the benefit of losing extra pounds. I'm sure Lisa has, as all good teachers do, has a lot of compassion for her students.

That year when Chris was working on his Eagle Scout project by collecting blankets, hats, scarves, and mittens for the Union Gospel Mission it turned out to be quite an experience for him. I remember your telling me how full the extra garage got as people donated jackets and boots as well.

The next generation seems to be learning compassion as well. Zack is a very sensitive ten year old. He recently had a "melt down" that they had too much food and so many didn't in the world. Grandma Pat took him grocery shopping for the food shelf. After the tsunami disaster in South Indonesia, his elementary school had a drive for relief funds. In one week they raised $3750.00. Zack collected $750.00, the highest of the students. I called him that night about bringing in that much money to school. He said, "I was so proud."

Grandma Pat took six year old Brooke shopping for supplies to send to needy children in foreign lands. First, they got plastic shoe box containers to fill for a local church. They bought various school supplies, toothpaste and brushes, bars of soap, and washcloths. Later when they were sorting the things out for each box, Brooke held up a washcloth to her body and said, "It wouldn't cover much."

Landon's youth group at Caledonia's United Methodist Church raised money for the local food shelf. Four boys were each given $40.00 to do the shopping after being reminded about making good food choices, nutrition, and food that could be on the shelf. When the boys unpacked their bags at the food shelf, they were all good choices, but they wondered when Landon pulled out of his bag a bottle of Mountain Dew and A&W root beer. The boys were questioned about their choices, and Landon, thirteen, replied with a smile stating, "Everyone needs a treat once in awhile."

When Emily, then thirteen, and Sharen were in China in 2001 they met Andy Zhou, a young sixteen year old Chinese boy, who spoke English very well. Andy became their volunteer interpreter. In the part of China where Andy lived the government provided education to only one child in a family. Andy made the decision at thirteen, that his younger sister should go to school, and he would continue learning on his own. After the girls returned they raised $2300 to get Andy back into school. They dressed in their Chinese clothes, brought some of the items they had bought in China, and made a presentation at the local civic clubs and their church. Family and friends also helped. Andy has just graduated from high school and is applying for college scholarships.

Compassion, caring, and kindness are traits all humanity should have. What a better place this world would be with more compassion for others. Do you remember when you first learned that you had breast cancer, how you didn't know anyone with it? Think back about how many you now know, and how much you have learned from them.

Peggy, your education and working experiences have prepared you for your fight against cancer. As a teacher you were always learning and researching. Now you are using those same skills to help others. I have learned much from you regarding breast cancer. The information that you sent me regarding the importance of diet and exercising to fight and lower the risk of cancer, brings me back to Mom's long remission. She always was physically active, we had balanced meals, no fast foods were available then. Mom always baked from "scratch." This may have contributed to those good years of 1936-1952.

In order to climb a mountain you have to go step by step. Fighting cancer is the same, step by step. To remain on top you must stay alert and watchful. Not wait until a crisis that knocks you down, like Mom did. I am guilty of the same. After my hysterectomy because of cancer, I never thought of cancer again. In the past thirty eight years I have had three pap smears and very few mammograms. I do go to the doctor often, but I can't remember when I had a physical. Fortunately, my kids aren't so careless.

Several years after Mom's death, Aunt Jeanette told me how Mom would pray after her first cancer operation. Every night she prayed to live long enough to see her children educated. This made me aware she may have known more than she let on. How proud she would be to have her first grandchild achieve her doctorate. Perhaps, this is something you will consider completing this fall.

I hope you remember what you learned about the toll emotional stress plays on your body. You have had more than one bad bout of cancer. What you learned, you must apply to your life to avoid a reccurrence. Your better eating habits and daily three mile walks are great. But don't be so "busy" and let others cause stress for you. Take time for yourself and enjoy the goodness of life.

228

Love,

Aunt Karen

P.S.

I've been catching up on my photo-scrapbooks. Usually a semi-annual job for me.

I added the tribute that was in the Duluth New Tribune-last October during Breast

Cancer Awareness month. Jim's a good and caring soul. God must have smiled when

you two met. In case you have forgotten his words, here they are:

"Peggy"

Margaret A. Anderson

"Four month survivor of breast and lymph cancer-retired teacher of grades 1-12,

parent, wife, and friend to many individuals. My wife has said many times that each

day is a beautiful gift and there are people who are far worse off in this world, and we

need to think of others and learn from them."

"Whether you irradiate or don't irradiate, whether you have lumpectomies or take the breast off, there is no difference for survival."

-National Surgical Adjuvant Breast Project

"Let your gentleness be evident to all.............."   -Philippians 4:5

"Trust in the Lord with all thine heart; and lean not unto thine own understanding. In all thy ways acknowledge Him, and He shall direct my paths."   -Proverbs 3: 5-6

"Better a meal of vegetables where there is love than a fattened calf with hatred."

-Proverbs 15:17

"Changes come from "I.""   -Author Unknown

"What the mind can conceive and believe the mind can achieve."   -Author Unknown

"Love comforts like sunshine after the rain."   -William Shakespeare

2/28/05

Dear Auntie,

Greetings! How's everything going? I enjoyed our conversation the other night about food. I do miss gourmet cooking.

I read about liver enzymes on the internet. Cancer patients can experience damage to their liver as a side effect to cancer treatment or to the spread of cancer in their liver. My doctor told me there are other reasons that enzymes go up as medication or weight related issues. Anyhow, I will be having them re-tested next week.

Jim and I are still busy going to the Center for Personal Fitness. Some of the men down there look like Supermen on steroids as they are constantly lifting weights. I wrote a story about why I go to the Center for Personal Fitness entitled, "Exercising is Like a Game of Chess" and changed it to "Exercising at the Center for Personal Fitness." I was a physical education major for four years, so I do know how important daily fitness is believe it or not. Back then I was a bean pole but as the stress of life got to me, I gained weight. I exercised my mind and not my body all these years.

There are many confusing messages about the foods we eat. I have learned it's better if you can get your sources of nutrition from your diet instead of supplements. How do we know we are deficient in anything? I guess we have to keep track of it in our upstairs attics. I've read so many different view points based on research, and maybe that's my problem, I read too much.

The *American Cancer Society* feels diet is very important and recommends eating five or more servings of fruits and vegetables a day. Fiber and water are very important as well. There are benefits from eating healthy as reduced diabetes, obesity, heart disease and a lowered risk for cancers. Watching your weight and not smoking are important, dear Auntie. As you can tell, cancer and nutrition winds me up!

The *International Agency for Research on Cancer* states that one-fourth to one-third of all cancers are attributed to being inactive and overweight. Fat effects weight in our bodies. I think of this one cartoon in an exercising book we bought, where a man is looking in a box of fat bundles, trying to figure out which bundle he should pick up and remove, like puppies in a box. I wish it was that easy for middle age women!

I wanted to tell you a little more about diet. A *Life Extension* health advisor recommended I take: indole 3, ketodhea, selenium, vitamin E, melatonin, and curcurmin each day. It was also recommended that I eat mushrooms (shittake). Well, I talked to my doctor about what I'm on, and she felt the indole 3, vitamin E, green tea tablets, fish oil, and multivitamins were fine but everything needs to be based on research. I told her my frustration in wanting to talk to someone locally as I showed her the book, *Beating Cancer with Nutrition* that listed the Duluth Clinic in the back. We discussed the blood tests that *Life Extension* recommended for hormone profiles. There are a lot of food books out there about cancer and nutrition, and I think I'll go to Barnes and Noble to look at a few.

One book is called *What to Eat if You Have Cancer* by Maureen Keane and Daniella Chace. I like this book because it is pretty clear cut and easy to understand. Another book, *How to Prevent Breast Cancer* by Dr. Pelton, Taffy Pelton, and Dr.

Vinton Vint is really excellent even if it's an older book. We need to take vitamin C, vitamin E, extra beta carotene, selenium, flaxseed oil, and coenzyme 10. There can be side effects from mixing drugs, and some cancer drugs may not be as effective with herbal drugs. But as you always told me, **discuss the pills with your doctor first.**

In the book *Beating Cancer with Nutrition* by Dr. Patrick Quillin, he tells the reader they need to have a good vitamin-mineral supplement, extra vitamin C, vitamin E, coenzyme 10, selenium, fish oil or chilled Norwegian cod liver oil, green tea extract, curcumin and conjugated linoleic acid. He feels our body removes toxins everyday. Dr. Quillin has a few quotes like," A well nourished cancer patient can better manage and beat the disease," and "There's convincing evidence that nutrition can change the way a body works." Dr. Quillin tells the listener on his tape how our bodies have packmen that gobble up the mistakes in the body. It makes you wonder why some people have better packman. In any case, our bodies are our disease fighting machines, Auntie.

Good nutrition is important to fighting cancer. We as a society have spent " fifty billion dollars on the 32 year war against cancer," according to Dr. Quillin. I think we need to look for our own answers in our bodies and environment. Dr. Quillin also tells us "optimal nutrition can cover quality and quantity of life." The cancer cells need to be stimulated for DNA repair. Our cells need antioxidation, protective enzymes and oxygenation to protect them from mutations. Phytochemicals are important to fight against cancer as well as antioxidants that promote healing by protecting the cells from free radicals, and they also slow the aging process. Phenolics have anti-tumor and anticancer properties. Flavonoids promote healthy growth and development of cells. Thiollyl boosts your immune system and helps the body to get rid of carcinogens. Indoles are necessary for healthy cells and to fight cancer. It's amazing that 42% of American get cancer and the rest fight it off in their bodies.

Thank you the other night for giving me this list of **anticancer foods. The ***

indoles are the cancer fighting foods. The others are good cancer protectors.
I'm typing these below so you can put it on your refrigerator to stay healthy.

Beverages: green and black tea

Fruits: apricots, cantaloupe, cranberries, red grapes, purple grapes, mangoes

Vegetables: artichokes, arugula, beets, bok choy, broccoli,* brussel sprouts,*
cabbage,* cauliflower,* carrots, green beans, greens (collard, kale, mustard, turnips,
romaine), onions, peppers (green red and hot), russet potatoes, radishes,* spinach,
squash, tomatoes,* turnips, *watercress, yams and sweet potatoes

Condiments: garlic, horseradish (fresh is better), mustard, sage,* turmeric *(used in
curry)

Fresh herbs: (mint, such as spearmint), rosemary.

I hope you liked the breast cancer diet plan in my other letter. You may want to
put this on your refrigerator because it is a way for you to eat healthy. There are a few
kinds of food I haven't heard of but I want to try.

We all have natural healing abilities when we have the system to fight it off.
Radiation, chemo and poor diet don't help in the cancer war. As patients we need
a healthy diet, which is our ammunition to fight this war. My immune system is
weakened from radiation and healing is little slow for me. I found that out when I had
my ears pieced in a few more places. You need to eat healthy to fight fungal infections.

I read the following information in a *Harvard Medical Report* on a cancer
prevention internet site:

Cancer Risk Factors	% of Cancer Deaths
Family history of cancer	5%
Diet (animal food based)	30%
Lack of exercise	5%
Smoking	30%
Carcinogens in the work place	5%

There was this interesting article on the internet about nutrition and the role it plays on all cancers, as well as breast cancer. It tells the reader that inappropriate food choices are thought to be the cause of 30-70% of all cancers. Our body is fighting a war on cancer every day of our lives. A strong immune system helps to wipe out cancer. Our body needs the correct nutrients as a computer needs power to run. I read on the internet that *breast cancer patients **should eat*** the following:

-**A good multivitamin**

-**Beverages**-(Avoid alcohol, caffeine and drinks containing stimulants. These drinks compete in removal of estrogen from the body, circulate the estrogen, and it becomes harder to excrete the estrogens.)

-**Cold water fish** (salmon, tuna, herring, mackerel, halibut)-These are all good choices of omega 3.

-Don't eat polyunsaturated fats or vegetable oils as corn, sunflower or safflower as they are associated with breast cancer. Instead use **olive oil**. (Petro's mom, from Athens, Greece, told Jim using olive oil was one way to lower his blood pressure years ago.)

-**Flaxseeds**

-**Fresh fruit** (cranberries)

-**Legumes**

-**Meats** (Eat no more than 3 oz. of meat a day or the size of playing cards. Avoid well done and burned meat because it your increases your cancer risk by five times. It's best to choose other choices of protein when possible or limit the red meat helpings. Hormones leave residue in the meat's fat and muscle. Antibiotics are found in the animal flesh as well. The fertilizers of the food that the animals eat contain heavy metals that has been found in breast tumors. Also pesticides and herbicides act as environmental estrogens.)

-**Organic vegetables** (broccoli, brussel sprouts, kale, mustard greens, cabbage)

-Sea vegetables

-Soy foods

February has ended with many activities. Many are the same, so I won't repeat them all. I've sure gotten a lot of cancer memories in my life. My thoughts and memories have filled a notebook as cancer has given me a new sense of purpose in life. Hopefully day by day, month by month, and year by year they will find the answer to breast cancer, so more lives can be saved in our community. To think that the American Cancer Society stated to me 1 out of every 7 women will get invasive cancer in their lifetime, and 1 in 10 African American women according to SEERS. It means that two people on both sides of my block will get it. Maybe we as patients have to find the answers in ourselves. I feel life is very precious, and I'm only going to have a healing spirit that says, "I can do this."

Our Radon test came back negative. Radon can cause cancer. I read in a book that it is important to not breathe paints, solvents, gasoline, pesticides, nail polish, glue, oven cleaner, and other household chemicals as it's bad for our cellular structure.

Also Petro's second wife called Lisa from Greece to ask the first wife a question. I thought this was interesting. I gave her my Lisa's phone number.

Life has changed the way I perceive things. I get bored easily so one day I made some breast cancer stationary to give away. I've given hundreds of dollars worth of books to Miller Dwan Foundation for the radiation library. As I did this, I thought of about Eileen and Paula Kochevar. Paula was my student at Lester Park Elementary School years ago. Eileen use to go to rummage sales a lot, and I would talk to here there. She use to be Faith Lutheran's secretary. I couldn't believe it a few years ago, when I asked our school librarian, Karen, about her. I was total shock to me that Eileen had died of cancer. She was such a wonderful person, and the radiation library was started because of her. I was so involved being a teacher that I lost track of what was happening in our community. In donating books I feel like I am doing something for the new cancer center that is being built no matter how small my part may be. We all need to do our part in this world. I have been extremely lucky to have such excellent doctors for my treatment (and staff). They are **some of the many** dedicated doctors (and staff) at the Duluth Clinic, Miller Dwan, and SMDC that give their heart and soul to their jobs everyday.

I'm also including a copy of my story with this letter about exercising, some complementary therapies for patients as well as people in general.

Love,

Peggy

Oh, I talked to a dietician at Miller Dwan, and she feels the 'New American Plate' approach from *The American Institute of Cancer Research* is the recommended diet approach for cancer prevention. I went to the website she recommended. We need to go from the old American plate to the new American plate. What is that? It's two-thirds of our plate should consist of vegetables, fruits, whole grains or beans. Animal protein would take up one-third or less of our plate. They also list on their website three strategies for cancer prevention. They are: 1.Eat a greater portion of plant foods. 2.Keep physically active and 3.Maintain a healthy weight. The same factors that apply to cancer prevention may also apply to preventing cancer recurrence after treatment. In general there has been very little research on the nutritional factors that influence cancer recurrence. The data is most compelling for breast cancer where the risk of recurrence might be increased by obesity, and diets high in fat and low in fruits and vegetables. Prostate cancer recurrence might also be increased by high saturated fat intake. Thus, it seems reasonable to recommend that cancer survivors follow the prevention guidelines outlined by the AICR.

Diagnostic Procedures and Complementary Treatments:

Acupuncture-This healing is based on penetrating the skin by electrical stimulation.

Alcohol-Women who drink need adequate amounts of folic acid (400-600) daily. Alcohol is not recommended for breast cancer patients.

Ayurveda-Diet and herbal remedies that use the body, mind, and spirit and have been used by the Indian culture for over 5,000 years.

Alternative Medical Systems-Systems build on theory and practice. They include homeopathic, naturopathic, Chinese traditional medicine and Ayurveda.

Animal Fat-Eating animal fat increases one's risk of breast cancer and research has documented this over and over. It causes more estrogen to be in the blood, so eat a low fat diet.

Anthocyanins-These are substances found in berries, yams, red grape skins, and citrus. Berries protect people from DNA damage, so eat plenty of these fruits, and as many colorful fruit and vegetables as you can.

Antioxidant System-A good antioxidant system prevents damage from oxidation.

Antioxidants-These chemicals are found in certain foods and are also produced in the body. They include vitamins A, E and C. Antioxidants protect the body against free radicals that alter your molecular structure in the complex process of oxidation.

Beta Carotene-This might help protect against cervical cancer as well.

Biologically Based Therapies-Therapies that are based on herbs, foods, and vitamins that are found in nature. They may include dietary supplements, herbal products and even unproven therapies.

Catechins-Substances found in berries, black and green tea help with cancer. protection. Drink caffeine free green tea as caffeine type products deplete your cells.

Cinnamon Capsules-These capsules have been used with people who have diabetes and have triglyceride problems. Always consult your physician first.

Chiropractic Care-A doctor that uses manipulative therapy on the bones of the body to align the body.

Cooking Meats-Cooking meat at 480 degrees on the grill or higher is thought to cause the formation of carcinogenic compounds called heterocyclic aromatic amines (HAA's).

Complementary Therapies- These are methods used to complement or to add to therapies to improve the quality of life for the individual cancer patient to lessen the physical and psychological side effects. They may include: acupuncture, acupressure, aerobics, affirmations, alexander therapy, American healing, applied kinesiology, anthroposophical medicine, aromatherapy, art therapy, ayurveda, biking, biography writing, breathing exercises or breath works, biofeedback, body works, bioenergetics, chiropractic care, committing to life activities, cranial therapy, crystals, cymatic therapy, dance therapy, essential oils, exercise, feeling therapy, feldenkrais method, faith healing, feng shui, grief therapy, guided visualization, holistic medicine, homeopathy, hydrotherapy, hypnosis hypnotherapy, hyperbaric oxygen therapy, humor therapy, journaling, kirlian photography, labyrinth walking, laser light therapy, light music therapy, macrobiotic diet, massage therapy, meditation, music therapy, Native American healing, naturopathy, neural therapy, neuro-linguistic programming, ohashiatsu, osteopathy, pilates, polarity therapy, prayer, psycho therapy, qo gong, reflexology or pressure points on the feet, rosen method, reiki, rolfing, scrap booking, self love therapy, shamanism, shiatsu, simple movements, skin stimulation, spirituality, support groups, tai chi, TCM, trayer approach, transcutaneous electrical nerve therapy, walking, writing briskly, and yoga.

Curcumin-(tumeric spice/curry)-A spice that has cancer fighting properties. It may repair DNA damage from radiation. It also protects against xenoestrogens as it can fit in the same receptors as estrogen. (Two studies have proven this but more are being done.) It's a powerful antioxidant that protects against free radicals.

Diet -A great diet for a breast cancer patient is one low in daily fat calories-low in caloric intake density-low in saturated animal fats-one that doesn't have lipid peroxide that destroys antioxidants-high in natural fiber grains, legumes, fruits, vegetables, and fish-carbohydrates are more complex-high in water soluble vitamins-foods that have vitamins C and B-lots of natural phytochemicals and antioxidants.

Energy Fields-These can be biofield therapies as Qi gong, Reiki, therapeutic touch, and bioelectromagnetic based therapies involving magnetic fields.

Exercise-Ideally walking 10,000 steps a day will effect diseases. A mile roughly 2,000 steps but use a pedometer. Other aerobics include classes, biking, running, balance training, and stretch exercises.

Folate-This nutrient occurs naturally in 150 different forms in nature. (ie folio acid, B vitamins can repair DNA.) Folic is destroyed by heat. Great raw sources of this are avocados, boysenberries, cantaloupe, alpha sprouts, broccoli and cauliflower.

Glucarates-These are found in fruits and vegetables and are important in boosting and detoxifying the immune system. (*Simone Protective Cancer Institute* did a study on these in 99' and found that 90% of all cancers are caused by dietary and nutritional factors.)

Homeopathic-Medicinal medicines used to cure or help diseases.

Hot Chili Peppers, Turmeric and Cumin-These seasonings are thought to prevent carcinogens from attaching to DNA and initiating cancer.

Immunotherapy-This is a way to enhance the body's immune system.

Indoles-Specific indoles are thought to fight against breast cancer. Breast cancer patients should eat broccoli, cabbage, brussel sprouts, turnips, kale, and dark leafy vegetables.

Iodine-Nori, kombi, and sea vegetables contain this mineral which protects against radiation. (Some feel our exposure to radioactive materials is strong in our environments.)

Isoflavonoids (Geinstein and Daidzen)-These deactivate excessive estrogen in your body and lower risk for hormone based breast cancer of the breast, cervix and

238

uterus. These food include soybeans, tempeh, misco, and very highly processed soy products. Estrogen positive women should discuss this with their doctors.

Integrative Medicine-Therapies that combine mainstream and medicine with CAM therapies.

Japanese Diet-This is a diet high in selenium, vitamin C and E that protects Japanese women from cancer. They also eat a lot of soy and phytoestrogens.

Ligans-Found in foods as flaxseeds and whole grains that block estrogen. It's thought that they reduce breast cancer.

Low Fat Diet-A low fat diet is very important for preventing breast cancer. Obesity alters liver metabolism, and you have higher estrogen by products. Obesity makes you insulin resistance and increases your sex hormone, SHBG, a bonding globulin.

Lycopenes-These are powerful arytenoids that reduce cancers. Examples are tomatoes, grapefruit, watermelons, and apricots.

Manipulative and Body Based Methods-Based on movement and manipulation of one or more body parts. These include chiropractor, osteopathic care or massage therapy.

Massage-A therapist stimulates muscle and tissue in the body.

Med Diet-This is a diet high in fruits, vegetables, whole grains, fish, nuts, olive oil, moderate red wine, low in meat and refined grains. One expert claims this diet will reduce breast cancer by 15%.

Metastic Cancer-There are more free radicals in this type of cancer that cause DNA damage. It's important to eat lots of antioxidants and vitamin C.

Naturopathy Treatment-This is mind and body medicine.

Mind-Body Interventions-These are techniques that enhance the minds ability to affect bodily functions and symptoms. Examples include mediation, prayer, mental healing, art, music, and dance therapies.

Monoterpenes-This helps prevent cancer by increasing the production of liver enzymes. It detoxifies the carcinogenic substances. An example is citrus fruits.

Naturopathic Medicine-A type of medicine that uses nutrition, counseling of life styles, dietary supplements, exercise, medicinal plants, homeopathy, and traditional Chinese medicine.

Nausea-Peppermint and ginger tea as well as pieces of ginger may help this problem.

Osteopathic Medicine-A type of medicine that uses manipulation of the full body to alleviate pain, restore body function, health, and well being of the patient.

Phytonutrients-These are cancer fighting foods and vegetables.

Phthalides-Anticancerous compounds found in celery, carrots and herbs. Other examples are parsley, dill, fennel, and corriander.

Processed Foods-Limit processed foods in your diet as they have many chemicals added.

Polyphenols-These are thought to lower the risk of breast cancer.

Protease Inhibitors-Foods that inhibit cancer. Examples are beans, potatoes, rice, and eggplant.

Proven Treatment Therapies-Evidence based, conventional, mainstream or standard medical treatment tested by strict guidelines, research based and approved by the food and drug administration.

Qi gong-Chinese medicine that combines movement, meditation and breathing to improve the immune function of the body and blood circulation.

Quercetin-This protects the body from DNA damage by inhibiting tumor stimulating enzymes and inactivating the cancer causing agents. Examples include shallots, red grapes, yellow squash, and broccoli.

Research or Investigational Therapies-Therapies used in clinical trials.

Reiki (Universal Life Energy)-Spiritual energy is used to heal the physical body.

Sulforaphanes-These are compounds that neutralize the carcinogens and speed up it's removal from the body. Examples are broccoli and cauliflower.

Sugars-Do not eat sugar other than natural sugar as it fuels cancer. Examples include: brown sugar, brown sugar syrup, corn syrup, dextrose, dextrin, fruit juices, high fructose, galactose, glucose, honey, hydrogenated starch, lactose, maple sryup polyols, sorbitol, raw sugar, and xylitol sucrose. Always read labels.

Tai chi-Mediation through breathing exercises.

Therapeutic Touch-Healing hands used to identify energy imbalances.

Traditional Chinese Medicine (TCM)-The concept of the balanced "chee."
A balance of the Yin (negative) with the Yang (positive).

Triterpenoids-This substance blocks estrogen and its ability to increase the risk of cancer. Examples are citrus fruits and soybeans.

Ways to Improve Your Breast Cancer Health-Monitor your body's burden by having the chemicals tested in your body. This can be done by blood tests, urine tests, and the milk of lactating mothers can be tested.

White Foods-Read labels and don't eat the following white foods unless you have to: bread, crackers, cookies, flour, rice, pasta, and sugar.

Medical Findings/Terminology:

Cancer Cells-Cells that cause DNA damage are called free radicals. Scientist are looking at ways that vitamins A, C, and E, as well as selenium protect people against cancer.

Chorline-Early studies have linked chlorine and breast cancer.

Citrus Pectin-Stimulates the immune system.

Coffee/Tea-Coffee and tea have antioxidants called polyphenols. Green, black, oolong tea retain polyphenols longer. Green tea has a protective mechanism against barrett's esophagus cancer and reflux disorders. It has catechins which is an anticancer food.

Deli Meats and Bacon-These are thought to be carcinogenic, possibly from nitrates.

Dietary Risk from an Environmental Working Group-There are 12 foods that we are at risk in eating due to pesticides and fertilizers. They are strawberries, peppers, spinach, cherries, peaches, cantaloupe, celery, apples, apricots, green beans, grapes and cucumbers. The site of orgins include the United States, Mexico, Chili, and other places.

Dietary Supplements-These include vitamins, minerals, and herbal supplements.

Diethylstibesterol and Dioxin-Toxins may be linked to breast cancer.

Electromagnetic Fields-Magnetic fields are believed to produce electrical currents from the earth's core.

Ellagic Acid-This is acid that stops cancerous cells and detoxifies carcinogens. It's found in fruits and vegetables. There's high quantities of it in apples, berries, cherries, grapes, and walnuts.

Feelings-Cancer patients are often critical of themselves, have experienced a loss of some sort, may have gone through a divorce, may have repressed anger and emotions, may have lost their home, maybe depressed, maybe self-sacrificing women, and could have sterile relationships with their spouses. Some breast cancer patients may need to address these feelings along with other feelings.

Fish Oil and Flaxseed Oil-These oils may inhibit cancer cells from attaching.

Glycemic Load-This is how much fat is in your blood and how sugar causes it to rise. Eat only foods to lower the glycemic load as beans, brown rice, fruits, lentils, whole grains, and vegetables.

Gylcemic Index-This effects the blood sugar on a fixed amount of food. If we add vinegar or lemon to a food with a high glycemic load it will reduce the load.

Isoflavonids-Weak plant estrogens are found in tofu, soymilk, soybeans, and soy products. They may be healthy for women who have normal estrogen ranges.

Ionizing Radiation-A type of radiation that has been linked to breast cancer when it occurs at crucial ages in a child's life or woman's life.

Immune Function-Antioxidants increase the fight against cancer by improving the immune function.

Nuclear Sources-These have long been known as a cause for breast cancer.

Nutrition-Food and growth repair tissue and the replacement of cells. Nutrition is what sets the stage for your body to fight diseases and you need a strong immune system.

Organic Food-These foods have no pesticides, no sewage baked fertilizers, petroleum food, genetic or radiation fertilizers when they were grown.

Organic and Free Range Animals -These animals would not have antibiotics and growth hormones injected into them. This goes for dairy products as well.

Pesticides-Women need to be careful on the produce they buy due to fertilizer and DDT exposure. High levels of DDT have shown up in women's malignant breast tumors.

Pomegrant Juice-This is a stronger antioxidant than red wine, blueberry juice, cranberry juice and green tea.

Salmon-Eat only wild salmon as it has fewer PCB's. Don't buy farm-raised salmon. Smaller salmon are safer than larger.

Vitamin A-An antioxidant that can weaken bones if you have excessive amounts. Don't take vitamin A supplements as it will interfere with the breakdown of old bone and can interfere with vitamin D which helps to maintain normal calcium levels.

Vitamin E-This vitamin can lead to small but noticeable increases in LDL and triglycerides.

Xenoestrogens-Environmental estrogens are given to cattle which settle in their fatty tissues.

Zinc-Zinc stimulates the immune system.

Life is like a game of chess. The rules of the game are called the laws of your body. Those who play the game well with the highest stakes win at the game of life. Those individuals who play poorly are checked with health problems and disease.

I have been checked with breast and metastatic lymph cancer. My primary tumor is estrogen/progesterone positive which means I can be treated by controlling the estrogen in my body. Estrogen is tied to circulating body fat by many sources. I have high triglycerides and cholesterol as well. According to a very large study by the American Cancer Society, it showed that sixty percent of women that were overweight were more likely to die from breast disease than normal weight women. There is information out there that has found two-thirds of women who are overweight develop breast cancer. Evidence shows that women who participate in physical activity may have protective effects from breast cancer if they are not obese.

Reports state that women with unusually high levels of estrogen can get estrogen dominance that sets the stage for cancer. Increased use of hormone replacement therapy puts high risk individuals at risk for breast cancer. Women should ask their doctors to monitor their hormone levels with blood tests. One in every seven women will get invasive breast cancer in their lifetime.

Alcohol also increases ones risk in the game. For example, if you have two drinks a day, the American Cancer Society states your risk is increased by 21% for getting breast cancer. Alcohol and other caffeine products are believed to increase estrogen circulation. A poor diet also sets the stage in this game that is played in life. A poor immune system allows your body to not have the tools to play the game. Education is important in playing chess well. You need to learn the rules to win. Those who play poorly lose.

I have played the game poorly by letting myself get overweight. Exercising everyday is something I do, so I can lose excessive fat that carries excessive estrogen circulating in my blood.

I don't want to be checkmated and be repeating the quote, "The Cancer of Life is Regret.: The rules of the game are clear. The ones who play the game right win. That's why you see me here often walking or on the treadmill.---Peggy Anderson

"In order to laugh, you must be able to play with your pain."   -Anette Goodheart

"Nine Essentials To a Full and Contented Life
   Health enough to work a pleasure.
   Wealth enough to support your needs.
   Love enough to move you to be useful and helpful to them.
   Strength to battle with difficulties and overcome them.
   Grace enough to confess your sins and overcome them.
   Patience enough to toil until some good is accomplished.
   Charity enough to see some good in your neighbor.
   Faith enough to make real the things of God.
   Hope enough to remove all anxious fears concerning the
   Future."   -Goethe

"God will never leave us nor forsake us."   -Hebrew 13:15

"Yesterday is history
Tomorrow is a mystery,
Today is a gift,
That's why we call it "the present."   -Unknown Author

3/15/05

Dear Auntie,

   This has been a busy last couple weeks with yoga classes, Breast Cancer Support group, seeing Dr. Seidelmann for a recheck, seeing my chiropractor, Dr. Torgrimson several times, soup suppers at church, and Bible study classes. Breast Cancer Support group had a meal provided by Heidi's Shop, and we saw all kinds of swim suits, scarves, and personal items. It was really fun as the nurse was very vivacious, and she let every one stay longer to talk.

   I got a stress fracture from walking three miles a day, so I'm in a cast for three weeks. I'm on calcium pills now, and I weigh 163 pounds on my weighted scale.

   Last Thursday I went to the second Spirit Team Board Meeting for the Breast Awareness program at the YWCA. Kim she is so full of energy. She was talking about the women she's known who have died of breast cancer, and how important it is to FIGHT the fight with courage. I will be telling you more about the first Spirit team meeting later on in this letter.

On Saturday I went to the Women's Expo 2005. I've never been to it before, and it's been going on in Duluth for ten years! Kim gave me a T-shirt, and I helped for an hour and a half. We recruited people for the Mother's Day Walk Run and tried to qualify women for free mammogram funding.

My personal paradigm has changed in many ways. I have had to do some soul searching to heal. I've been on an emotional roller coaster over this breast cancer wake up call and trying to find the cause of my cancer with some certainty. Causes are not that black and white. I've had to learn a lot of medical jargon and fill my brain with information that was totally unfamiliar to me. I read in a book called *Breast Cancer Answers* by Judy King about the risk factors, and they are as follows:

1.Genetic or related risk factors: (family history, perinatal factors/growth, reproductive, prescription drugs/medical procedures) account for 14% of all cancers.

2.Environmental Risks: (viruses/other biological agents, pollution, ionizing/ultraviolet radiation) account for 9% of all cancers.

3.Lifestyle Risk Factors: (tobacco, adult diet/obesity, sedentary lifestyle, occupational/ job related factors, alcohol, socioeconomic status, salt-food additives and other preservatives/contaminants) account for an amazing 77% of all cancers. This is pretty amazing statistics!

Food--I thought it was interesting awhile back when you told me, we shouldn't eat more than a deck of cards of protein per day. Wow, that's not very much, and we were eating 2-3x's that per supper meal.

I want to tell you more about the YWCA Spirit Team Board that I am on. We've had two meetings, and I think it's going to be a lot of fun being involved with breast cancer awareness activities. Kim is so energetic and dynamic. She has made amazing things happen in Duluth with her energy and guidance. At the first meeting, Kim said she had to talk to legislators about health insurance caps for breast cancer women. I can't believe in this day and age some women will have to go without treatment and pills because of a $5,000.00 cap on Minnesota Care. The doctors perform surgery on women, and they are sent out there to die because of lack of follow up treatments and pills.

Kim gave me a couple of booklets. One I found especially interesting was by the Breast Cancer Fund/Breast Cancer Action entitled: *State of the Evidence-What is the Connection Between the Environment and Breast Cancer?* This booklet said, "Research indicates that breast cancer arises for four primary reasons: genetic mutation, altered gene expression, altered cell interaction or from exposure to agents that alter the body's natural production of estrogen and other hormones." We get cancer from a number of exposures. It goes on to explain in the next paragraph, "In addition, compelling scientific evidence points to some of the 85,000 synthetic chemicals in use today that are contributing to the development of breast cancer, either by altering hormone function or gene expression. As with ionizing radiation, some synthetic chemicals (called mutagens) also cause gene mutations that lead to breast cancer." This means there is evidence that chemical exposures and breast cancer have a link. Women with a predisposition are more sensitive to these carcinogens, and we need to be better educated to what they are. This book also tells of how " the Women's Health Initiative Study on Hormone Replacement Therapy was halted when it became clear that women who regularly took HRT (hormone replacement therapy) had significantly higher rates of breast cancer." It also goes on to state that "*The National Toxicology Program* now lists steroidal estrogens as known human carcinogens." This is not new, as *the International Agency of Research on Cancer* states the same thing. Hormones have a value, yet they can be a double edged knife for the potential cancer patient. I'm enclosing a list of substances listed in the *U.S. National Toxicology Program's 10th Report on Carcinogens* that are known causes of mammary tumors. She talked to me about Jamie Harvie, who is very knowledgeable about toxins, and I made an appointment to see him.

Thanks, Auntie, for the good news on breast cancer research from the National Jewish researchers. It was interesting how women with normal breast cells have relatively high levels of cdk6, whereas women with breast cancer cells have low levels to nonexistent levels of cdk6. Sounds like to prevent breast cancer this cdk6 needs to be kept up in women, so malignant cells won't divide. The National Jewish Center may have found a valuable marker for breast cancer and a way to target the control of cell growth.

There is a Mother's Day Walk Run for Breast Cancer in May. My Lisa said she would walk with me. There's also the Relay for Life at St. Scholastica during the year put on by American Cancer but my church is not going to have a team this year as many individuals work the next day. Duluth also has the Dragon Boat Festival which is a rowing race to raise funds for non-profit organizations as United Way, Red Cross, and American Cancer. I guess they select a different organization each year. They have an organization called Survivor Sisterhood that participates by having a team, and I saw the race on television one year.

My Lisa was over and read our first letters in my notebook. She asked, "Do you own a forest? She saw all the paper piled high on my dining room table that I'm using for a makeshift desk. She's surprised that I wrote this book from our letters. Lisa probably thought I had constipation of the brain and couldn't get it out. Jim is anxious for me to go on to a new project. My dear husband feels I've neglected him by not feeding him gourmet meals, cleaning the house, and giving him my undivided attention. He thinks I'm stuck on the breast cancer chapter of my life and wants to see me move on. Jim doesn't realize how important it is for women to know the causes of breast cancer and try to make changes in their lives. Too many women are getting breast cancer. We need answers!!!

Love,

Peggy

"Today is the first day of the rest of your life!"   -Unknown Author

"All the flowers of Tomorrow, are in the seeds of Today."   -Chinese Proverb

"Goodness is the only investment that never fails."   -Unknown Author

"Happiness won't find you. You have to find it."   -Unknown Author

"Yesterday is but a dream, tomorrow is only a vision. But today, well lived, makes every yesterday a dream of happiness, and every tomorrow a vision of hope. Look well, therefore, to this day, for it is life, the very life of life."   -Sanskrit Proverb

"But small is the gate and narrow the road that leads to life, and only a few find it."
                                                                    -Matthew 7:14

4/5/05

Dear Auntie,

From the lens of my eyes this has been a tough year. My soul and life have been through many seasons. I now look back, survived breast cancer, and learned how to cope. Things could be a lot worse as Kim's friend had a seven centimeter tumor under her arm. Just think March 21st was the first day of spring. Now we can look forward to all the summer and outside activities.

I can see what was on the blank page of my notebook. I went from seeing nothing on the page to seeing words that helped me to get better. I went from only being able to do small tasks to doing bigger tasks. I have gone from thinking I would never see the light of day, to seeing the sunset and rise with vibrant colors. I have gone from doing one thing to seeking a daily balance in my life. I have gone from not knowing how to handle daily stress, to putting it all in a place where I can process it, and move it away through meditation and prayer. I have gone to extensive conversations with my Maker. I have gone from being overweight to losing weight and feeling better in my mind about myself. I have gone from a blank CD to wonderful sound clips in mind while listening to so many CD tapes as I walk. I have gone from not feeling, to feeling much. I look at the world through all my many senses now. I think I have a balanced approach to my healing and thinking.

In the midst of life, I see the road back to normal. It's one you need to trudge lightly on, and an individual always needs to keep focused on their goals. I wanted to document what I went through, how I struggled to find the answers, and a way to help our daughters by writing our letters. All this may help others in our community understand the struggle we go through as breast cancer survivors. It may help them to have hope, courage, endurance and be brave. Cancer has changed my life. I have learned new medical language, met a network of new people that are a part of my medical team, have had a lot of appointments, met other breast cancer survivors and listened to their stories, and I look at life differently.

Lots of busy times these last few months. Many church activities as well as Spirit Team meetings. I stopped by Central High School to see Wendy, and we had a discussion about benign tumors. She was telling me how she saw somewhere that 8 out of 10 tumors are benign. We sure need to know that as women, so we don't worry. I stopped at the clinic recently to see Lisa Starr about my frustrations about putting this all into a book. She's always so positive on the outside. I don't know how these medical people do this day after day. They are truly the heart and soul of the Duluth Clinic, and we have to give them a whole lot of credit.

I have come to know some wonderful people in my life because of something tragic, namely cancer. I have learned it is not a bad thing to get your priorities in order. Cancer can be a gift in that it is a wakeup call to our bodies. It can teach us to live with grace and kindness towards all other human beings. If we live with God's plan, we should look forward to the time we have on earth in our temporary temples. All the goodness of all the tomorrows and what we can do while here is important. God wants all of us for something better than this life. With this in mind, I can't help but think, we all need to do our very best for each other.

Karen, I wanted to tell you I called my second cousin, Bobbi, the other night about our family breast cancer history. I was shocked to learn at least seven Meier descendants have had cervical cancer. Ovarian cancer is a hereditary marker. Isn't this interesting. Bobbi said great Aunt Clara died of breast cancer, her mom had two fibrosis, and she had one with surgery. In correspondence with her I found out she had cervical and endometrial cancer that involved one ovary. Terry had cervical cancer as well. Bobbi's sister, Terry, died at age 36. (Terry was large breasted, size 44. She may have had dense breasts, if large breasted.) Her stage II breast cancer had metastasized, in spite of having chemo and radiation. Oh, Bobbi is in the Duluth Clinic Star Program. Terry had her age against her as do younger and older women. They now say AMAS testing, tomography, ultrasound, and breast MRI's should be used as mammography doesn't pick up fast growing tumors in dense breasted women. I'm a living example of that.

I saw Dr. Torgrimson, my chiropractor, this month. I asked him about the quote he stated to me last time. It was "Inch by inch anything is a cinch" by Robert Schuller. I had my back and neck adjusted and inch by inch I'm getting better.

On the 23rd I met with Jamie Harvie, who I had talked to on the phone several times. He's a Duluth man who is very knowledgeable about toxins and cancer. We discussed how we all have a body burden, and that breast tumors and body fat contain toxins. (I did read that mothers who breast feed pass these toxins on to future generations. If mothers don't breast feed they are at risk for breast cancer. Ironic!) We discussed the role of hormones in one's body. Jamie said that hormones may get confused when they try to attach to a receptor, as he showed this with his hand movements. I told him I take Armidex to block my receptors and take vitamin E and fish oil to make the receptors slippery. Jamie said toxins may have estrogenic type properties. He cited an interesting example that it's like putting a house key into a car engine. We've all tried that. He gave me a card with six actions on it to reduce exposure to cancer causing chemicals and environmental hazards from the Breast Cancer Fund. I've attached this because it's easier to understand.

Another time when I talked to Jamie, we discussed a public health perspective being different from a clinical treatment perspective. The medical profession deals with treatment, or the results as the cancer. The public health community wants to know the causes, and they want the government to control the causes. Jamie cited how we recognized twenty years ago that smoking more than likely caused cancer, but we couldn't prove it until recently. I told him I knew what he meant. Then I pointed out to him that I feel the new SMDC Cancer Center in Duluth will have a more holistic approach to healing. I went on to tell him patients are a wealth of information about what has happened to them. We just need to be asked the right questions!

Then we discussed the *State of the Evidence* booklet that says there is strong evidence that breast cancer is caused by exposure to estrogens, DES, and ionizing radiation. There also is good evidence linking breast cancer to aromatic amines, found in the plastic and chemical industries, in tobacco smoke, and grilled meat and fish. Chemicals such as benzene and ethylene oxide are also associated with increased risk of breast cancer. As I left Jamie's office, I told him I was writing a book. I didn't tell him about my health minor and strong interest in health. Jamie is a very interesting, knowledgeable community resource and I was glad to have the opportunity to chat with him.

We can reduce our risk of breast cancer by choosing a healthy diet, minimizing alcohol consumption, not smoking, getting regular exercise, breastfeeding our children, and avoiding hormone replacement therapy when we reach menopause. We can improve our chances for early detection of breast cancer by doing breast self examinations, having an annual clinical breast examination (beginning at age 20) and having an annual mammogram (after age 50). Free mammograms are available to qualifying women. Women who are 50 years old or older have the greatest risk of breast cancer but all women should be vigilant in monitoring their health. We can't control our genetic makeup--so women with a strong family history of breast cancer or ovarian cancer need to make their primary physician aware of this special vulnerability. We can control some environmental exposures by buying only organic produce, for example, and by limiting consumption of red meat and dairy products (which may contain hormones), avoiding pesticide use at home, and by minimizing the use of certain plastics, particularly for microwaving and storing food. But everyday we're exposed to hundreds of chemicals in the air, food, and water, as well as electromagnetic fields in the home and workplace. Reducing or eliminating those exposures will require chances in public policy to protect our health.

On the 30th I met with Dr. Krook, my oncologist, and I want to tell you more about this appointment. I had blood work and a mammogram before seeing him. My mammogram is probably benign, Birads 3 and looks good. My blood tests are normal except for the same ones that are an issue (liver enzymes, cholesterol, and triglerides.) I go back to see Dr. Krook in three months. I asked Dr. Krook how a person could tell if they had metastasis and he said, "You wouldn't be eating, you'd be losing weight, and you could have pain or a growth." This summed it up real well. He reminded me that I chose to not do chemo. I told him I didn't want to because of the many side effects. I told him about my 2nd cousin dying of stage 2 breast cancer that metastasized. He said it can happen with stage one. I was thinking cancer is a strange phenomenon. It acts and can reoccur for no rhyme or reason. Terry had all the treatments, and she died. I think our best bet in all this is to go to our doctors, be persistent to any body changes, and build up our bodies defense mechanisms. We have to be positive each day. So many women have beaten the odds. Doctors can't be held responsible for such vigilance in the body. We as patients have to look for the signs, go to the doctors, and demand tests if we have concerns.

Dr. Krook is so funny, so smart. I sometimes get lost in his exampling certain things that I ask him. Some of this medical jargon is " Greek to me." I can't believe this doctor who knows this dance with death is so overly positive. Humor is great therapy, and he is a doctor that really demonstrates this.

I'm going to unpack a few more boxes in the attic from last fall. The packrat is still in me, but I'm going to sort through our belongings. We don't need all this stuff.

I don't want to have the light bulb go off in my head, as I look frantically for missing items I can't find. I've made too many lists. This brainstorm in my head has been swirling for too many years working over time, and it needs a rest. I want to use figments of my creative imagination to do the things that give others pleasure in life before I'm gone. Maybe that's God's plan for me.

I'm thinking about hope, looking at the past and present, as I do a time travel of this past year and my purpose here on earth amidst my potpourri of remembrances. Some of these thoughts have changed in size, color, and the way they look. The fish gets bigger, I suppose. I know we all have a strong purpose based on a higher spiritual power. There's peace in my life, my soul, and I can deal with whatever is in store for me down the road. I want to go back to graduate school, but I don't know about the stressors. Should I do things I have a deep rooted passion for or lose this opportunity to go back. This is the last year I have to go back to teaching in Duluth after retiring. Should I go back part time? If it's meant to be it will happen. I continue to express how I feel. I often live for the moment, but can do more long term tasks as writing this book. Will I ever be able to bury breast cancer in my trunk upstairs like other memories? (Well, this is my song and story.)

It's been a year since I felt my breast lump. This month I had my cast off, but have to be careful of my right heel. If I get a stress fracture again, I'll be in a cast for a lot longer time. Dr. Lillegard said I can't do strenuous walking for two weeks and then I have to build up to it as he laid out a plan for me to follow.

I met with Dr. Park Skinner on the 31st about the small, almond shaped lump under my breast. She removed it and was it gross like chicken fat. She thought it was a lymphoma, as did Dr. Krook and Dr. Nisswandt. Anyhow, it will no longer be rubbing under my bra.

At breast cancer support group this month we had Jody, a music therapist from St. Mary's, do some therapy activities and she did a great job! We also got information about the Susan G. Komen Breast Cancer 3-Day Walk and the Dragon Boat Race for

Survivor Sisterhood.

We didn't make it to the Empty Bowl, maybe next year. Jim had to work at Feast of Nations for Police Reserves. Next year I'm going to go to it with someone. There are many activities we haven't gone to in Duluth. Everyday there's so much on the calendar, I'm always busy. To think that I retired on 6/6/03, took 30 graduate credits, got burning problems in my chest, got breast cancer, had three surgeries, radiation and hormone therapy, and have just completed this book. I wrote this all down, so other women in our community will know what a woman goes through, what symptoms to look for, and to find a book loaded with information that could be helpful. You know my frustration about trying to find details in so many books and on the internet. I see why women give up.

I think about 1 out of 7 women getting invasive breast cancer on my block. We need to work to educate women on the causes of breast cancer, the symptoms of breast cancer, how to be look for signs that cancer has spread, so cancer can be treated early, and to help our communities to get all the diagnostic and treatment machines for breast cancer. As women, we need to write to our legislators to change health insurance, so it covers all types of breast cancer diagnostic tests, and monitoring tests. We need to make changes in our own lives, so that we can see if these changes can make a difference in the number of deaths occurring from breast cancer. Only by being active in our communities will our voices and cries be heard, and the cure will be found. We need to fight the fight with courage, faith, hope, the will to live, and a determination to make change.

I talked to my Lisa about "the book". She said, "I thought you were going to be done with breast cancer this year?" If it were that easy. Oh, Helen and I will be going to a formal tea at the Duluth Women's Club in a few weeks. Hope all is well with with you. Life goes on but call when you get a chance.

Lovingly,

Peggy

Follow up 106-Reoccurrences and Other Treatments Choices
Cancer Facts, Terms, Knowledge, and Concepts

Cancer Terminology:

Aneuploid Cells-These are the abnormal amounts of DNA, and if you have this it will be a more aggressive cancer.

Apoptosis-This is cell death failure.

Blood Tests-These tests tell the patient if the cancer prevention is working, the status of their immune system, and protein storage.

Bone Marrow Aspiration-This is the removing of bone marrow to stage cancer.

Breast Cancer Spreading-Breast cancer spreads by way of the lymph glands, lymph nodes, and blood. It can spread by the axillary nodes (under the arm), cervical glands (in the neck), and supraclavicular nodes (above the collar bone).

Bone Density-This is the bone resorption rate.

Bone Scan-This test can pick up cancer, stress on bones and joints.

Cancer Symptoms-dry mouth, eating issues, fatigue, nausea, sick feeling, sore mouth, sore throat, and tiredness

Colony-This is a stimulating factor. It shuts down when your blood count is too low.

Complan/Build Up-High calorie drinks for those who need them.

Dana Farber Research-There are 21 genes on a cancer cell, and they have found that looking at these they can determine if you need chemo.

DPD (Deoxypyridinoline Urine Test)-This is a test that tells bone absorption rates.

Diploid Tumor Cells-These cells contain normal amounts of human genetic material, DNA. If you have this it is a more favorable prognosis.

Distant Metastatic Disease-A new tumor is "distant." It can go into the bone, liver, lungs, spine, and brain. If it goes into these places the cure rate is low.

  Also it can go in to the lymph nodes and also reoccur on skin tissue.

Distant Reccurrence-Cancer comes back in the bones, brain, lung, live, or spine as shortness of breath, chronic cough, weight loss, and bone pain.

Dry Mouth-Use alcohol free mouth wash, drink sugar free drinks, put olive oil on the lining of your mouth before bed to keep it moist.

DXA-Bone scan.

Gene Signature Research-A Pokeman gene in the future may help in treating cancer.

Her-2/neu (c-erb B12)-This onogene leads to the development of cancer. If you have high levels of this, you may be resistant to hormone therapy as well as some types of chemo.

Life Time Risk-If someone in your family has cancer, you have a life time risk of getting cancer that could be 35-85%. Often both breasts removed are your best protection by several sources.

Local Reccurrence-This is when the cancer comes back at the lumpectomy or mastectomy site.

Megace (Megestrol Accetate)-These are steroids that boost your appetite.

Metastasizing-This is the spreading of cancer from the original tumor to other distant locations to grow by way of the lymphatic system, lymph nodes, and blood system. There are areas that it often goes to and they include the lung, liver and bones.

Metastatic Disease-As tumors grow they metastasize abnormal cells. Ten percent of the women with tumors smaller than 1 cm. will have metastasis breast cancer. Tumors that are 5 cms or larger will metastasize. They can also go into the lymph nodes, underarms and neck.

Micrometastases (Micromets)-These are cells that grow secondary tumors in the lymph nodes, bones, spinal cord, lungs, and liver.

MRI-This is a test that can pick out cancerous tumors.

Nano Shells-Rice University is doing a study to determine future breast cancer versus chemo.

Not Hungry-Eat light calories, eat natural fresh foods, at nutritional supplements as recommended by your doctor.

Nausea-This can be caused from radiation, radiotherapy, chemo, painkillers, infections, constipation, irritation to the stomach lining, and bowel blockages.

Nausea Treatment-The doctor may prescribe antiemetics. Sometimes complementary therapies work as acupuncture, homeopathy, imagery, medication, relaxation, yoga and visualization. Avoid certain foods as fast foods, fatty foods and foods that have a strong smell, and avoid hot foods. Small snacks or smaller meals work. Drink liquids slowly and with a straw but don't drink too much before a meal. Sea bands or acupressure wristbands sometimes work.

Oncotype DX-The first oncology test that uses gene expression of a patient's tumor to see if the invasive cancer will reoccur.

PET Test-This is a test that can tell cancerous tissues from normal tissues and scar tissue.

Primary Tumor-This is where the cancer starts.

QCT Bone Test (Quantitative Computerized Tomography/QCT Densitometry-This is a test that should be done annually which measures bone mass.

RAS Mutations-These are oncogenes that govern the regulation of cancer cell death.

S-phase Fraction-This is on a 1-25 scale. This is the percentage of cells that are dividing into the tumor. It's the cell cycle in which the DNA is replicating or making copies of itself. This new set goes into a new cell. If the results are seven percent or greater this is favorable. If the cells are immature cells they may be more aggressive. A high percent of cells means more rapid growth.

Secondary Tumor-This is the second site of a tumor or where the tumor part has gone to.

Sore Throats-The doctor may prescribe an antiseptic mouth wash or have you take a painkiller. Clean your teeth after each meal using a soft tooth brush, use baking soda if tooth paste bothers you and use dental floss gently. Eat pineapple chunks for juice. Use Vaseline or lip balm that is safe on your lips if they are dry. Add gravy and sauces to your food to make them more liquid. Avoid tobacco, hot spicy foods, garlic, vinegar, salty foods or spices. Drink 8 glasses of water a day which can include

256

herbal tea, weak coffee, and sugarless, natural fruit juices. Suck on ice cubes or use a straw. Use an anesthetic gel and painkillers if directed by your doctor.

Trust in Mouth-Get an antifungal medicine.

Tumor Suppressor Genes-These are genes that stop tumors from forming.

Survival Rates For a Five Year Period: According to one source it is….

Breast Cancer that is localized-97%

Breast Cancer that has spread to the lymph nodes-79%

Breast Cancer that has spread to distant sites-23%

Survival Rates for More Advanced Cancer-Women can survive with the same quality of life with the new therapies, if given the correct treatment on time. It's up to the patient to go in when there are symptoms.

Tiredness-Accept help from others, do what you can do, exercise some, keep active, make changes in your life, plan each day, and do things in small steps.

Ultrasound-This is a good test for liver metastases.

Xeloda-This is an oral chemo for metastasis breast cancer.

Appendix

Chemicals Shown To Induce Mammary Tumors In Animals

(National Toxicology Program, 2003)
http://ntp-server.niehs.nih.gov/htdocs/Sites/MAMM.html

- Acronycine
- Benzene
- 2,2-BIS(Bromomethyl)-1,3-Propanediol
- 1,3-Butadiene
- 2-Chloroacetophenone (CN)
- Chloroprene
- C.I. Acid Red 114
- C.I. Basic Red 9 Monohydrochloride
- Clonitralid
- Cytembena
- 2,4-Diaminotoluene (2,4-Toluene Diamine)
- 1,2-Dibromo-3-Chloropropane
- 1,2-Dibromomoethane
- 2,3-Dibromo-1-Propanol
- 1,1-Dichlorethane
- 1,2-Dichlorethane
- 1,2-Dichloropropane (Propylene Dichloride)
- Dichlorvos
- 3,3'-Dimethoxybenzidine Dihydrochloride
- 3,3'-Dimethylbenzidine Dihydrochloride
- 2,4-Dinitrotoluene
- Ethylene Oxide
- Furosemide (Lasix)
- Glycidol
- Hydrazobenzene
- Indium Phosphide
- Isophosphamide
- Isoprene
- Methylene Chloride
- Methyleugenol
- Nithiazide
- 5-Nitroacenaphthene
- Nitrofurazone
- Nitromethane
- O-Nitrotoluene
- Ochratoxin A
- Phenesterin
- Procarbazine Hydrochloride
- Reserpine (Serpasil)
- Sulfallate
- 2,4- & 2,6-Toluene Diisocyanate
- O-Toluidine Hydrochloride
- 1,2,3-Trichloropropane
- Urethane
- Urethane and Ethanol Combination

SIX ACTIONS

to reduce your exposure to cancer-causing chemicals and environmental hazards!

For more details on these six actions or to view scientific sources for any of these facts, contact the Breast Cancer Fund.

TOLL FREE
1-866-760-TBCF

E-MAIL
info@breastcancerfund.org

WEB
www.breastcancerfund.org

MAIL
1388 Sutter St., Suite 400
San Francisco, CA 94109

1

Practice Healthy Purchasing

Don't bring toxic chemicals home from the store. Choose chlorine-free paper products to reduce dioxin, a carcinogen released when chlorinated products are incinerated. Read food labels, and choose pesticide-free, organic produce and hormone-free meats and dairy products. Replace harmful household cleaners that contain bleach with cheaper, nontoxic alternatives like baking soda, borax soap and vinegar. Look for alternatives to chemical weed and bug killers—many contain toxic chemicals that accumulate in our bodies.

2

Advocate for Safe Cosmetics

Chemicals linked to cancer and birth defects do not belong in cosmetics, period. However, some popular brands of shampoo, deodorant, face cream and other everyday products contain these dangerous chemicals. Join us in our demand for safer products and smarter laws by letting cosmetics companies know they need a makeover. Ask them to sign the Compact for Safe Cosmetics, a pledge to substitute chemicals linked to birth defects, infertility, cancer, brain damage and other serious health consequences with safer alternatives. Because we all have a right to safe and healthy personal care products.

3

Use Caution with Plastics

Some plastics leach hormone-disrupting chemicals called phthalates into the substances they touch. Polyvinyl chloride (PVC) plastics release carcinogens into our air and water during the production process. PVC plastics are especially dangerous in toys that children put in their mouths, so keep an eye out for nontoxic toys. Further, never put plastic or plastic wrap in the microwave, as this can release phthalates into your food and beverages.

4

Advocate for Clean Air

The soot and fumes released by factories, automobiles, diesel trucks and tobacco products contain chemicals called polycyclic aromatic hydrocarbons (PAHs) that are linked to breast cancer. Indeed, breathing these compounds from secondhand tobacco smoke may increase your risk for breast cancer more than active smoking. Stay away from secondhand smoke, and advocate for stronger clean air protections.

5

Avoid Unnecessary Radiation

Ionizing radiation is a known cause of breast cancer. Radiation damage to genes is cumulative over a lifetime—thus many low doses may have the same effect as a single high dose. Mammograms, other X-rays and CT scans expose you to radiation. While mammography screening may benefit postmenopausal women, mammography for women in their 30s and 40s remains controversial. Whenever you have an X-ray or scan, request a lead shield to protect the areas of your body not being X-rayed.

6

Explore Alternatives to Artificial Estrogens

Women who have prolonged exposure to estrogens are at higher risk for breast cancer, and major studies continue to show an increased risk when postmenopausal women use hormone replacement therapy (HRT). Women who use both birth control pills and—later in life—HRT face an even greater risk of breast cancer than those who use neither. Explore your options with healthcare professionals.

Symptoms of Recurrence/Metastasizing Cancer

Breast Cancer Metastases:

Breast cancer moves from the breast to the lymph nodes before it goes elsewhere. It often goes to the liver, bone, lungs, brain or spinal cord.

25% shows up in the bone
20% shows up in the lungs
25% shows up in the liver
Less frequently brain and spinal cord

These are criteria and **tests** the doctor can use to determine how aggressive your cancer is, and how likely it can metastasize, or has metastasized in determining your prognosis.

Information:	Better Prognosis	Not as Good Prognosis
Kind of cancer or tumor type	DCIS, LCIS, tubular, papillary medullary, colloid	infiltrating ductual (1 or more), infiltrating lobular (1 or more), inflammatory
Histologic Grade of cancer (1-3)	Well differentiated of low grade or highly differ grade 1is good. Moderately differ grade 2 is not bad.	Poorly differentiated of high grade means chemo and ovarian ablation.
Axillary Nodes	Negative lymph nodes are a good sign (no cancer)	Positive lymph nodes are not a good sign. (Cancer), high levels of capthepsin D are likely to have recurrences

260

Estrogen/ Progesterone Receptors (ER/PR Assay)	Positive nodes can be treated with hormone blockers.	Negative nodes can't be treated with hormone blockers. Chemo and ovaries removed.
HER-2/neu oncogene	Negative or absent is best.	Positive or . present is worse.
Stages of the Cancer	0-2 is the best	3-4 is the worst
P53	Negative or is absent the best.	Positive or present is the worse.
DNA Content	Diploid is the best.	Aneuploid/haploid is the worst.
S Phase	Less is better	High S fraction, means aggressive
Margins of the tumor	Clear is best.	Dirty or residual is more involved
Cell examination	Smooth margins Normal nuclei Mass	Jagged edges Big nuclei Dead cells in center
Tumor size (Primary)	Less than 1.5 is better	More than 1.5 is worse
Cycling Index	Less cell nuclear antigen present, and proliferating	More nuclear antigen and proliferating is worse.

__Bone Cancer Symptoms__:
The patient can't sleep due to bone pain, bones are brittle and fracture easily as the cancer eats up all the bone spaces as pressure is applied to the bones, and over the counter medicines no longer work on the patient.
Tests to diagnosis bone cancer:
-bone scans, x-rays, CAT scan (Computer Axial Tomography), MRI, PET, bone density tests as DPD, QCT, DEXA
__Treatment__: Radiation, Chemo, Hormone Therapy, Radiotherapy, Radioisotopes, bone injections

----

__Lung Cancer Symptoms:__
The patient has shortness of breath, chronic cough, and can't sleep.
Tests to diagnosis lung cancer:
-chest x-ray (difficult to see), needle biopsy, PET
__Treatment:__ Chemo

__Liver Cancer Symptoms:__
The patient will have weight loss, fever, anorexia, gastrointestinal trouble, or pain on right abdomen side.
Tests to diagnosis liver cancer:
-blood tests, liver scan, CAT, ultrasound tests, CT test, x-ray, PET
__Treatment:__ Surgery, chemo

__Brain/Spinal Cord Cancer Symptoms:__
The patient may have headaches, double vision, unbalanced walking, neurological symptoms, and does not feel well.
Tests to diagnosis brain/spinal cord cancer:
-MRI of brain, spinal cord, abdomen, PET
__Treatment:__ Radiation

__What Should You Report to Your Doctor?__ balance problems, bone pain, breathing problems as shortness of breath, bumps, chronic cough, headaches, lack of appetite, new lumps, pain, redness on the cancer site, weakness, and weight loss.

__Graver Cancer Signs:__ bleeding, cancer that is 2 inches long, cancer that is attached to the chest wall, cancer that doesn't move, hot and red skin at the cancer site, large lymph nodes under the arm or above the collar bone, ulcerated areas on the skin, and swollen fluid filled areas.

Monitoring Cancer by Blood Tests and Other Tests: **(Some tests maybe monthly, or every 3-6 months.)**

Anemia Test (Hepatic Dsyfunction)-This is a test that can be effected from cancer.

Chem Screen (SMAC)-Indicates if your liver and bone enzymes are normal.

CBC-This is a complete blood screening, and it tells if you have anemia or are iron deficient.

White Blood Cell Count (WBC's)-WBC counts indicates your body's immunity in fighting infection.

Red Blood Cells (RBC's)-These are the cells that carry oxygen to all the body parts.

Blood Tumor Marker Study-This is a blood test that measures the tumor in the blood, and a high count indicates a possible reccurrence of cancer.

Parathyroid Hormone Test-Another marker test.

CA 125-This test is a blood tumor marker test that can signal secondary breast cancer.

CA 27.29- A blood tumor test you could have every 3-6 months to detect cancer reccurrence. It does not detect early stage cancer. Non-cancerous conditions can elevate the blood as well. Not all cancers show up in the blood.

CA 15.3-This is a sensitive blood tumor marker for primary, preoperative and metastatic breast cancer. It names the protein in the breast cancer.

CEA (Carcinoembryonic Antigen)-This is a marker for secondary breast cancer. Small amounts are present in patients with a wide variety of cancer types. Other diseases can cause it to go up as well.

Creatine-Kinase BB-This is a marker for breast cancer.

Estrogen and Progesterone-These are female hormones, and doctors can have your tumor tested to see if it is positive, so you can be treated with hormone blockers.

GGTP-Another blood test.

Her 2/neu-If you test positive for this, your cancer will grow quickly.

Liver Enzyme Tests:

-1.AST-Liver Enzyme Test (SGOT-Serum Glutei Oxaloacetric Transaminase)
Your liver rearranges the building blocks of protein and damaged liver cells are released into the blood.

-2.AFP-Found in liver cancer cells.

-3.GGT-A marker for liver cancer.

P 53 Gene Mutation-This p53 protein is a tumor suppressor from the p53 gene. It acts as a guardian to DNA. If you get this mutation, it blocks abnormal cell growth. People who have one functional copy of p53 from a parent are predisposed to cancer in adulthood.

Prolactin-Another test.

Ras Mutation-Inhibition of Ras protein is important. Ras induces the expression of MDM2 gene, whose protein inhibits the p53 protein activity.

Serum Calcium Levels-This is a test that measures the increased calcium which could indicate bone cancer.

Testing for Angiogenesis-Woman who have 100 or more new vessels have reccurrences in 3 years according to a study.

TRUQUANT-This is another tumor marker test for breast cancer.

Urinary test-Women with metastasizing cancer have elevated urinary concentrations of fibroblast growth factors after surgery.

Other tests:
Full body scans-can detect early cancer, but there are risky levels of radiation.
Other tests-PET, CAT

Survival Rate Information:
Survival Rates for Localized Breast Cancer according to the American
Cancer Society Cancer Facts and Figures 2005:
5 years-98%
10 years-69%
15 years-15%

Survival Rates for Regional Metastatic Breast Cancer to the Nodes:
5 years-80%
(Prognosis for distant metastatic breast cancer depends on hormone receptor status, HER-2/neu status, location and extent of the disease, the period time a women is disease free, the metastatic recurrence, as well as other medical conditions prior treatment, response to the treatment, and age of the patient.)

Survival for Very Distant Metastases:
5 years-26%
After this it declines

Relative Survival Rates:
According to the 2003-2004 Breast Cancer Facts and Figures..
- "Based on the most recent data, **relative survival rates** for women diagnosed with breast cancer are:
-87% after 5 years of diagnosis
-77% after 10 years;
-63% after 15 years
-52% after 20 years"

Age At Diagnosis Survival Rates:
According to the American Cancer Society (2003-2004 Facts and Figures)…"*Age at diagnosis*-"For women under 40 years of age with breast cancer, 5-year relative survival rates are slightly lower, which may due to their tumors being more aggressive and less responsive to hormonal therapy.
-83% for women ages 45 and below;
-87% for women ages 45-54;
-88% for women ages 55-64

-89% for women ages 65-74;
-88% for women ages 65 and over;
-86% for women ages 75 and over"

Final Choices: There are many choices to make in regards to your final death. These may include a will, a living will, hospice care, euthanasia, planning your funeral, donating your body or body parts.

Cancer Occurrences:

The American Cancer Society states that...
-"Breast cancer is the **second leading cause of cancer** death in women."
-"Currently a woman living in the U.S. has a 13.4% or **1** in **7**, lifetime risk of developing breast cancer. However, a larger portion of the overall lifetime risk is due to the risks at older ages."
-"An African American Women has a 1 in 10 life time risk of getting invasive breast cancer."
-There is "an estimated **211,240 new cases** of invasive breast cancer are expected to occur in women in the U.S. **in 2005**."
-"In addition to invasive breast cancer, 58,490 new cases of in situ breast cancer are expected to occur among women during 2005."
-"Carcinoma in situ (CIS) accounts for about 58,490 new cases each year."
-"**In 2005**, about **40,410 women** and **460 men** will die from breast cancer in the United States."
-"According to the most recent data, mortality rates declined by 2.3% per year from 1990 to 2001 in all women, with larger decreases in younger (-50 years) women."

The National Cancer Institute states that...
-Breast cancer is "the leading cause of death among women ages 40-59."

The National Center for Health Statistics (our national database) states that....
-There were "1,702,577 deaths from breast cancer between the years of 1950-2001 (52 years)." This information comes from death certificates.

Information from the Minnesota Susan G. Komen Breast Cancer internet article dated 9/9/04 states...
-"The majority of all breast cancer occurs in women with no known risk factors."
-"All women are at risk-one's risk increases with age."
-"Life time risk (by age 85) of developing breast cancer is 1 in 7."
-"The best opportunity to reduce mortality and increase treatment options is through early detection."
-"Mammography is the best known method of early detection."

American Cancer Society for Minnesota statistics state that...
- "Breast cancer accounts in Minnesota for 1 out of every 3 cancers."
-"In Minnesota, 48% of women who have breast cancer will be 65 years of age or older, 31% will be 50-64 years of age and the remaining 21% will be 49 years of age or below."
-"Breast cancer is greatest among white women in Minnesota with blacks leading second."

-"Breast cancer is highest in Minnesota in the metro areas of Hennepin and Ramsey counties due to the socioeconomic base."

__American Cancer Society__......(2003-2004 Breast Cancer Facts and Figures)
-Obesity….. "A recent large American Cancer study showed that overweight women are 60% more likely to die from breast cancer compared to normal weight women."
-HRT……"Use of combination estrogen and progestin HTR increases a women's risk for breast cancer."
-Alcohol Consumption… "Alcohol is the dietary factor most consistently associated with increased breast cancer risk." - "The most likely mechanism is by which alcohol increases risk of breast cancer is by increasing estrogen and androgen levels"
-Physical Activity…."The available evidence supports a small protective association between physical activity and breast cancer."

Five-Year Relative Survival Rates* by Stage at Diagnosis, 1995-2000

Site	All Stages %	Local %	Regional %	Distant %	Site	All Stages %	Local %	Regional %	Distant %
Breast (female)	87.7	97.5	80.4	25.5	Ovary†	44.0	93.5	68.8	28.5
Colon & rectum	63.4	89.9	67.3	9.6	Pancreas	4.4	15.2	6.8	1.8
Esophagus	14.3	29.3	13.3	3.1	Prostate‡	99.3	100.0	–	33.5
Kidney	63.9	91.1	59.1	9.3	Stomach	23.3	58.4	22.5	3.1
Larynx	65.1	83.7	48.7	18.7	Testis	95.9	99.4	95.9	71.8
Liver	8.3	18.4	6.2	2.9	Thyroid	96.5	99.6	96.3	61.0
Lung & bronchus	15.2	49.4	16.1	2.1	Urinary bladder	81.7	94.1	48.8	5.5
Melanoma	90.5	97.6	60.3	16.2	Uterine cervix	72.7	92.2	53.3	16.8
Oral cavity	58.7	81.0	50.7	29.5	Uterine corpus	84.4	95.8	67.0	25.6

*Rates are adjusted for normal life expectancy and are based on cases diagnosed from 1995-2000, followed through 2001. †Recent changes in classification of ovarian cancer, namely excluding borderline tumors, has affected 1995-2000 survival rates. ‡The rate for local stage represents local and regional stages combined.

Local: An invasive malignant cancer confined entirely to the organ of origin. **Regional:** A malignant cancer that 1) has extended beyond the limits of the organ of origin directly into surrounding organs or tissues; 2) involves regional lymph nodes by way of lymphatic system; or 3) has both regional extension and involvement of regional lymph nodes. **Distant:** A malignant cancer that has spread to parts of the body remote from the primary tumor either by direct extension or by discontinuous metastasis to distant organs, tissues, or via the lymphatic system to distant lymph nodes.

Source: Surveillance, Epidemiology, and End Results Program, 1975-2001, Division of Cancer Control and Population Sciences, National Cancer Institute, Bethesda, MD, 2004.

American Cancer Society, Surveillance Research, 2005

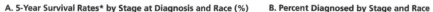

Figure 8. Female Breast Cancer – United States, 1992-1999

A. 5-Year Survival Rates* by Stage at Diagnosis and Race (%)

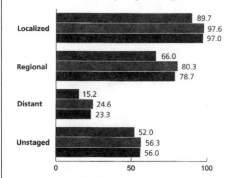

	African American	White	All Races
Localized	89.7	97.6	97.0
Regional	66.0	80.3	78.7
Distant	15.2	24.6	23.3
Unstaged	52.0	56.3	56.0

B. Percent Diagnosed by Stage and Race

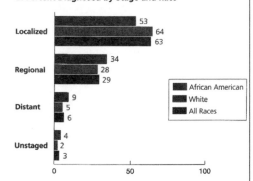

	African American	White	All Races
Localized	53	64	63
Regional	34	28	29
Distant	9	5	6
Unstaged	4	2	3

*Survival rates are based on follow-up of patients diagnosed between 1992-99 and followed through 2000.

Data source: Surveillance, Epidemiology, and End Results Program, 1973-2000, Division of Cancer Control and Population Sciences, National Cancer Institute, 2003.

American Cancer Society, Surveillance Research, 2003.

Table 2. Estimated New Breast Cancer Cases and Deaths in Women by Age, United States, 2003

Age	In Situ Cases*	%	Invasive Cases*	%	Deaths*	%
<30	100	0.2	1,000	0.5	100	0.3
30-39	2,100	3.8	10,500	5.0	1,300	3.3
40-49	12,600	22.6	35,500	16.8	4,300	10.8
50-59	15,700	28.2	48,700	23.0	7,000	17.6
60-69	11,500	20.6	43,100	20.4	7,400	18.6
70-79	10,100	18.1	45,600	21.6	9,500	23.9
80+	3,500	6.3	27,000	12.8	10,100	25.4
Total	**55,700**	**100.0**	**211,300**	**100.0**	**39,800**	**100.0**

*Rounding to nearest hundred
Percentages may not exactly total 100%, due to rounding.

American Cancer Society, Surveillance Research, 2003.

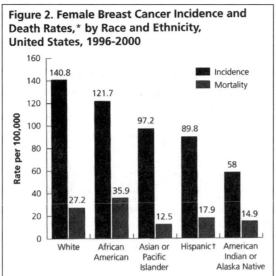

Figure 2. Female Breast Cancer Incidence and Death Rates,* by Race and Ethnicity, United States, 1996-2000

Rate per 100,000

Race/Ethnicity	Incidence	Mortality
White	140.8	27.2
African American	121.7	35.9
Asian or Pacific Islander	97.2	12.5
Hispanic†	89.8	17.9
American Indian or Alaska Native	58	14.9

*Rates are age-adjusted to the 2000 US standard population.
†Persons of Hispanic origin may be any race.

Data sources: *Incidence* – Surveillance, Epidemiology, and End Results Program, 1973-2000, Division of Cancer Control and Population Science, National Cancer Institute, 2003. *Deaths* – National Center for Health Statistics, Centers for Disease Control and Prevention, 2003.

American Cancer Society, Surveillance Research, 2003.

Table 1. Female Breast Cancer Incidence and Death Rates* (1996-2000) by Race and State

State	White Incidence†	White Mortality‡	African American Incidence†	African American Mortality‡	State	White Incidence†	White Mortality‡	African American Incidence†	African American Mortality‡
Alabama	§	24.6	§	33.3	Montana	133.9	24.8	§	¶
Alaska	146.0	25.9	147.6	¶	Nebraska	130.5	25.3	121.7	41.8
Arizona	123.9	25.7	95.6	33.2	Nevada	§	26.9	§	32.2
Arkansas	§	23.7	§	37.4	New Hampshire	§	28.2	§	¶
California	140.9	27.6	119.4	34.9	New Jersey	143.1	31.2	115.7	37.2
Colorado	137.5	24.1	99.3	36.0	New Mexico	122.3	26.1	94.4	40.2
Connecticut	144.4	27.5	115.7	33.1	New York	135.5	30.4	99.3	32.3
Delaware	§	29.7	§	39.1	North Carolina	124.6	24.9	111.2	36.2
Dist. of Columbia	§	27.4	§	42.6	North Dakota	§	26.6	§	¶
Florida	133.7	25.0	103.4	31.9	Ohio	128.5	29.1	117.1	38.6
Georgia	§	25.1	§	34.2	Oklahoma	§	26.7	§	38.8
Hawaii	152.1	27.1	§	¶	Oregon	143.4	26.8	121.5	29.7
Idaho	129.9	26.6	§	¶	Pennsylvania	130.1	29.0	116.2	37.7
Illinois	134.2	29.2	121.8	39.9	Rhode Island	135.7	29.7	89.8	27.4
Indiana	§	27.7	§	40.0	South Carolina	§	24.8	§	36.4
Iowa	130.6	26.4	128.8	37.4	South Dakota	§	25.3	§	¶
Kansas	§	25.5	§	40.1	Tennessee	§	26.0	§	37.0
Kentucky	122.8	26.8	127.6	35.7	Texas	§	25.2	§	37.1
Louisiana	124.4	27.3	114.2	38.2	Utah	118.7	23.8	40.3	¶
Maine	§	26.5	§	¶	Vermont	§	27.4	§	¶
Maryland	§	28.3	§	35.5	Virginia	§	27.1	§	38.2
Massachusetts	§	29.0	§	27.5	Washington	146.7	26.0	114.1	38.6
Michigan	132.1	27.3	121.4	36.9	West Virginia	119.9	27.4	115.9	42.5
Minnesota	137.8	26.7	104.2	34.5	Wisconsin	132.1	26.5	116.1	30.7
Mississippi	§	24.8	§	37.4	Wyoming	126.6	26.6	§	¶
Missouri	§	26.3	§	37.1					

*All rates are per 100,000 and age-adjusted to 2000 US standard population.
†Source is SEER and NPCR areas reported by the North American Association of Central Cancer Registries as meeting high quality standards for 1996-2000.
‡Death data are from CDC's National Vital Statistics System and cover the entire US population (http://www.cdc.gov/nchs).
§Statistic could not be calculated because state did not submit data to NAACCR, meet quality standards, or had six or fewer cases.
¶25 or fewer deaths; statistic could not be calculated.

American Cancer Society, Surveillance Research, 2003.

Probability of Developing Invasive Cancers Over Selected Age Intervals, by Sex, US, 1999-2001*

		Birth to 39 (%)	40 to 59 (%)	60 to 79 (%)	Birth to Death (%)
All sites†	Male	1.41 (1 in 71)	8.52 (1 in 12)	34.63 (1 in 3)	45.59 (1 in 2)
	Female	1.97 (1 in 51)	9.10 (1 in 11)	22.51 (1 in 4)	38.18 (1 in 3)
Urinary	Male	.02 (1 in 4264)	.41 (1 in 243)	2.42 (1 in 41)	3.56 (1 in 28)
bladder‡	Female	.01 (1 in 8876)	.12 (1 in 804)	.65 (1 in 153)	1.13 (1 in 88)
Breast	Female	.48 (1 in 207)	4.18 (1 in 24)	7.49 (1 in 13)	13.39 (1 in 7)
Colon &	Male	.07 (1 in 1484)	.90 (1 in 111)	3.96 (1 in 25)	5.90 (1 in 17)
rectum	Female	.06 (1 in 1586)	.69 (1 in 145)	3.04 (1 in 33)	5.54 (1 in 18)
Leukemia	Male	.15 (1 in 659)	.22 (1 in 461)	.85 (1 in 118)	1.47 (1 in 68)
	Female	.13 (1 in 799)	.14 (1 in 697)	.48 (1 in 206)	1.04 (1 in 96)
Lung &	Male	.03 (1 in 3164)	1.06 (1 in 95)	5.75 (1 in 17)	7.63 (1 in 13)
bronchus	Female	.03 (1 in 2977)	.81 (1 in 123)	3.91 (1 in 26)	5.71 (1 in 18)
Melanoma	Male	.13 (1 in 795)	.51 (1 in 195)	1.08 (1 in 93)	1.89 (1 in 53)
of skin	Female	.21 (1 in 484)	.40 (1 in 248)	.53 (1 in 190)	1.28 (1 in 78)
Non-Hodgkin	Male	.14 (1 in 724)	.46 (1 in 217)	1.32 (1 in 76)	2.18 (1 in 46)
lymphoma	Female	.09 (1 in 1147)	.31 (1 in 328)	1.00 (1 in 100)	1.80 (1 in 56)
Prostate	Male	.01 (1 in 9879)	2.58 (1 in 39)	14.76 (1 in 7)	17.81 (1 in 6)
Uterine cervix	Female	.16 (1 in 636)	.29 (1 in 340)	.27 (1 in 368)	.77 (1 in 130)
Uterine corpus	Female	.06 (1 in 1632)	.72 (1 in 139)	1.57 (1 in 64)	2.62 (1 in 38)

*For those free of cancer at beginning of age interval. Based on cancer cases diagnosed during 1999-2001. The "1 in" statistic and the inverse of the percentage may not be equivalent due to rounding.
†All sites exclude basal and squamous cell skin cancers and in situ carcinomas except urinary bladder. ‡Includes invasive and in situ cancer cases.
Source: DEVCAN: Probability of Developing or Dying of Cancer Software, Version 5.2. Statistical Research and Applications Branch, National Cancer Institute, 2004. http://srab.cancer.gov/devcan

American Cancer Society, Surveillance Research, 2005

Grief Stages That A Breast Cancer Patient Must Work Through

A patient must work through the following stages:
1.Denial/Shock
2.Anger/Fear
3.Sadness/Why Me?
4.Acceptance

1.Denial (State of Shock)-A breast cancer patient denies they have cancer, and they have to work through the sudden shock of owning the situation placed upon them. Why has this happened to them? Or it's not happening to them, they feel numb, or they feel they are losing control in their lives. The patient is placed in a state of crisis and doesn't want to deal with it because of the shock.

2.Anger or Fear-The patient may feel angry at God, the world, themselves, and who ever is in their immediate surroundings. The fear of not knowing how they got breast cancer may be overwhelming. Part of the anger could be transferred to the fear of the unknown. What did they do to deserve this? What did they do wrong? Will they live or will they die?

3.Sadness (Why Me?)-A more deep rooted sadness and grief may occur. The patient may feel isolated, depressed, unhappy, helpless, singled out, be unable to go on with their daily activities, feel like a higher power has failed them, and the patient could feel deeply troubled with "the why did this happen to them." Why were they chosen?

4.Acceptance-The patient has learned to accept their disease and may have had to talk to someone. There is a sense of resolve and renewal in what has happened to them as they reconstruct their previous way of life, maybe looking at it in a new way. Breast cancer no longer owns them as they are participate fully in life. They looking forward to many good days.

After Thoughts: Looking At My Past, Present, and Future

At the time of this publishing, I am cancer free or in remission. I know this can change. As a breast cancer survivor, I read cancer reports and treatments as they come out in the news or in magazines, and search for any change in statistics. A cancer patient's biggest fear is recurrence.

This book was an inspiration when I asked my Auntie, Why Me? It became a reality when I put it into a book. My hopes is that it will be useful to my daughter, my cousins, my nieces, and the readers of this book. I tried to write a book that would appeal to all types of readers: those who like true stories by way of letters for the holistic right brain reader/ learner; facts, information, and charts for the left brained/ analytical reader/learner; pictures and print for the multi sensory reader/ learner. Some of the many pictures and cancer information were afterthoughts to our letters.

Cancer can be a life shattering and upsetting experience because of fear of the unknown. My feeling is that education is power, and if we know how our enemy works (or the disease) we can fight the fight! It's so important to understand all there is there is about this disease, so we can be our own best advocates, look at the "Why did this happen?," "How it can be prevented?," as so many women have recurrences later in life according to their death certificates.

The road back to happiness can be painful but it is happier on the other side. There are many women out there that spend years grieving over breast cancer and their lose. In talking to other women, I realize it is so important to treat breast cancer patients with a holistic approach, so they can move forward through the grief stages that they experience. I see as I go through my book that I have gone through these stages. It's important to get to the other side of the rainbow, to the pot of gold. If I look back, I've had cancer several times, and I'm still alive. This life has been a blessed and fruitful life, thanks to my family, friends, the people I've come to know, and my teaching career. I look forward to my future as well, thanks to the many wonderful doctors and medical personnel.

MEET MY AUNTIE

Karen Prahl McDonald is my Father's sister. She lived in Duluth until 1974 when the Burlington Northern Railroad transferred Uncle Jim to Minneapolis where they make their home in Brooklyn Park. Karen is the mother of three children and grandmother to six. She is very proud that each of her children has chosen a career that serves others. Sharen, her oldest is a social worker. Nancy, the youngest is in her 16th year of teaching and Jeff, her middle child, is a therapist who recently changed from working with troubled juveniles to a new challenge of helping families in need.

My aunt and I have always had a special bond of love and keep in close touch with letters and phone calls. We are strong and unwavering supporters of each other.

In 1999, Karen was diagnosised with Chronic Obstructive Pulmonary Disease (COPD) after years of various lung infections. She's been on corticosteroids for more than ten years because of asthma, chronic bronchitis and emphysema health problems. In the summer of 1999 she had the opportunity to join a Lung Power Rehabilitation Group at Unity Hospital to learn how to live with this disease. At age 77 she still goes two mornings a week to exercise and to consult with her case managers, except when she's battling one of her many bouts of pneumonia, broken ribs, or repeated lung fungal infections.

Her philosophy of life can be best summed up by the following story she sent me several years ago…"The Fork"

The Fork

There was a woman, Doertta Jakoby, who had been diagnosed with cancer and had been told there was nothing more they could do for her. So she contacted her pastor and had him come to her house to discuss certain aspects of her final wishes. She told him which songs she wanted sung at the service, what scriptures she would like read, and what she wanted to be wearing. The woman also told her pastor that she wanted to be buried with her favorite Bible.

Everything was in order and the pastor was preparing to leave. When the woman suddenly remembered something very important to her.

"There's one more thing." she said excitedly.

"What's that?" came the pastor's reply.

"This is very important." the woman continued. "I want to be buried with a fork in my left hand and my Bible in right hand."

The pastor stood looking at the woman not knowing quite what to say.

"That shocks you, doesn't it ?" The woman asked.

"Well, to be honest, I'm puzzled by the request," said the pastor.

The woman explained. "In all my years of attending church socials and functions where food was involved, my favorite part was when whoever was cleaning away the dishes of the main course would lean over and say, "You can keep your fork." It was my favorite part because I knew that something better was coming. When they told me to keep my fork, I knew that something great was about to be given to me. It wasn't just jello or pudding. It was cake or pie, something with substance. So I just wanted people to see me there in that casket with a fork in my hand and I wanted them to wonder "What's with the fork?" Then I want you to tell them: "Something better is coming, so keep your fork too."

The pastor's eyes were welted up with tears of joy as he hugged the woman good-bye. He knew this would be one of the last times he would see her before her death. But he also knew that the woman had a better grasp of heaven than he did. She KNEW that something better was coming.

At the funeral people were walking by the woman's casket and they saw her in a beautiful wedding dress she had worn when she married Mike, her favorite Bible in her right hand and the fork placed in her left hand. Over and over the pastor heard the question "What's with the fork?" And over and over he smiled. During his message the pastor told the people of his conversation he had with the woman shortly before she died. He also told them about the fork and about what it symbolized to her. The pastor told the people how he could not stop thinking about the fork and told them that they probably would not be able to stop thinking about it either. He was right.

So the next time you reach down for your fork, let it remind you, oh so gently, that there is something better coming. Not just in death but in life as well.

-Author Unknown

MEET MY AUNTIE
with her fork!
(A great aunt, friend,
spiritual advisor and
counselor!)

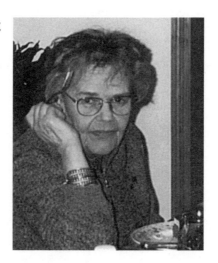

There are several things you can do to help yourself.

1.Find the cause(s) of your cancer.

Life Extension in their literature states that 60% of breast cancer patients are estrogen positive. Take hormone blockers as prescribed by your oncologist, as estrogen attaches to receptors, and it's energy fuel for some cancers.

Watch weaker estrogens if you are estrogen positive. They may increase the estrogen in your body. More studies are being done on phytoestrogens and the jury is still out on this issue. (Foods that contain phtyoestrogens are apples, asparagus, barley, beans, blackberries, bok choy, carrots, cereals, cherries, corn, dried seaweed, fennel, flaxseeds, garlic, green pepper, kale, legumes, licorice, milk, mustard greens, oat bran, oats, olive oil, onions, pears, pomegranate, radishes, soy products, squash, sunflower seeds, wheat germ, and yams.)

Be careful with environmental toxins like xenoestrogens, excessive radiation, and other household toxic chemicals that cause excessive stimulation and DNA damage to breast tissue. Our body already have a body burden of toxins. We carry these around with us until death, as all toxins are not excreted by the body!

2.Rebuild your power by improving your immune system.

Look at your immune system and change your diet by cutting off the enemies energy supply line. A quality diet helps your body to build your fighting warriors, so foods with additives and chemicals can't effect you.

Eat plenty of fruits and vegetables that are colorful and rich in antioxidants throughout the day. Choose vegetables from the cabbage family that are full of indoles. Sugar fuels cancer in a breast cancer patient, so only eat natural sugar as it is in fruit. Be more aware of labels and what's in products.

Eliminate or cut down on red meat. A lot of red meat, some poultry, and some dairy are laden with hormones and pesticides. Choose organic beef and hormone free poultry. If you eat regular beef, limit the amount and chose fat free cuts. (This advice is for estrogen positive women who are overweight.) Organic or low fat dairy is a wise decision as well. Eat more fish but chose smaller fish from large fresh oceans. Fish should be free from mercury and PCB's. Don't eat salted, cured, smoked meats with nitrates in them.

Grains, fiber, legumes are important, so eat unprocessed grains. Plenty of fiber every day is important to rid your body of estrogen. Legumes can be a good protein source as well.

Drinking plenty of fluid is important for cellular structure and growth. Caffeine dehydrates the bodies cells as does alcohol. Caffeine free choices are best when drinking tea. Good choices could include bottled water, natural fruit juices (sugar free), V-8 juice, Bolt house, Green Tea and Naked Juices.

Limit the spices to those that are anticancer spices. Use olive oil and butter over other choices.

3.Environment is important.

Sunlight is important as it boosts the immune system but don't sunbathe. Spend the day breathing in clean air.

Control your environment by getting rid of toxic people and avoiding toxic environments. Watch what you do on high ozone days depending on where you live, if you have allergies, and asthma.

Don't put pesticides on your lawn, use natural cleaning products in your home, and don't buy products with PVC, phthalates, biphenyl A and other dangerous chemicals in them.

4.Attitude is important.

A healthy attitude with positive affirmations promotes positive thoughts. Find out what's stressing your body, reduce the stress and stressors by letting the feelings out, and controlling your environment if necessary. Find peace within you and in the world.

Be in charge of your life. Get copies of your medical records to keep informed, as knowledge is power. Research your options, beat the odds.

5.Help yourself by empowerment.

Gather personal strength through optimism and hope. Improve your self esteem by feeling good, looking good, and doing good works.

Peel back the onion, and look at each layer in the core of your strengths. Address your strengths, and make your own life style changes, stop smoking and drinking, listen to music, pamper yourself, laugh often to improve your endorphins, enjoy life and people, experience life through all your senses (touch, taste, feel, hearing, and sight).

Have a sense of reverence through prayer and spirituality. Seek a spirit of balance in all that you do. Faith sometimes seems like it is being tested, and it is a humbling experience when you feel it's being tested by the Almighty here on earth.

Think of others and help them by being thoughtful, being kind, offering a helping hand, caring, being cheerful, being concerned, and looking at what they have to offer. Ask yourself: What can you done for someone else?

Motivate others to strength by celebrating life with a merry heart. Endorphins are brought on by happiness that stimulate the immune system. Your first three years can bring the highest chance of recurrence. Motivate others with your strength.

Look for joy and lasting fulfillment in life by celebrating life everyday!

Fight the fight for life. Tell yourself--"I can do this." " I will help myself and others in this world." "Leave this world by making a difference in other people's lives."

How To Help In Your Community and Make The Breast Cancer Fight Known

1.Volunteer and be part of breast cancer activities in your community. In Northern Minnesota there's The Breast Awareness Program (Duluth, MN),- Encore Programs (in various cities)-Mother's Day Walk-Run (Duluth, MN)- Dragon Boat Festival Race (Survivor Sisterhood Group, Duluth, MN)- The Relay for Life (American Cancer-in most towns and cities), and Susan G. Komen 3 Day Walk (Minneapolis).

2.Be an advocate for someone else who has cancer by following your heart. It may be notes, positive affirmations, cards, a meal, or even a ride.

3.Raise funds for breast cancer in your community. (ie-medical facilities that have breast programs, American Cancer, and Encore Programs.)

4.Be a mentor to someone with breast cancer. Volunteer to do things with them or remember the individual in small memorable ways.

5.Donate books on breast cancer or cancer to your local cancer facilities and breast awareness programs in your community. (ie-Miller Dwan Foundation for the new Cancer Center. Donate used or new breast cancer books, home made gifts, prizes, prosthesis, wigs and other recycled breast cancer items to your local Encore programs.)

6.Send for free breast cancer materials and make them available in your church or in nursing homes. Speak at your church or at a nursing home about breast cancer.

7.Join a breast cancer support group and try to build public awareness of the issues involved with breast cancer. Also find out what communities and boards you can be on in your community to build breast cancer awareness.

8.Be a political activist by write letters to your congressmen. (ie-Contact your local American Cancer as they has issues they want addressed. Breast cancer and cancer organizations need support!)

9.Donate money to programs in your community that can make a difference in breast cancer education, training, purchasing diagnostic and treatment equipment. (ie-Miller Dwan Foundation (education, training, equipment), SMDC Foundation (education, training, equipment), American Cancer (research and causes of breast cancer), and the Duluth YWCA Encore Breast Program (education).)

Miller Dwan Foundation
502 E. 2nd St.
Duluth, MN 55805

SMDC Foundation
400 E. Third St.
Duluth, MN 55805

American Cancer Society (local)
130 W. Superior St.
Duluth, MN 55802

American Cancer Society (Minnesota)
2520 Pilot Knob Rd. Suite 150
Mendota Heights, MN 55210

American Cancer Society(National)   YWCA Breast Awareness Program
1599 Clifton Rd. N.E.   202 West 2nd ST.
Atlanta, GA 30329   Duluth, MN 55802

10.Have your church make and donate **breast cancer scarves to your local cancer radiation and chemo facilities.** (ie-to the Duluth Breast Awareness program, Duluth Clinic Oncology Program, and Miller Dwan Radiation.)

"That best portion of a good man's life-His little, nameless, unremembered acts of kindness and love."   -William Wordsworth

Don't let cancer own you, defeat, cripple or destroy you. It doesn't have to be a death sentence, as there are nine million cancer patients alive in this world today. You can battle the war and win like so many others. Build your immune system up and fight back the war with the strongest force you have. Own the cancer and control the cancer.

Don't let cancer eat at your soul and being. Get rid of the personal demons that eat away at you. Control your advice, and get rid of being number one. God's tears are gifts and a part of life. Be the victor by climbing the ladder you know best up to the top.

Don't let cancer change your priorities in life. Everyone and everyday has full potential so draw on those strengths. Go on with your life with full force, enthusiasm, self-renewal, and determination. Make a difference in this world, as you have much to live for and offer. Seek a commitment of excellence for a job well done in this life by being an icon of strength through touching the lives of others. These are the only gifts that really matter in this life.

Cancer can't kill your memories, friendships, conquer your spirit, heart or soul. It teaches you to not waste precious moments in time. Cancer tells you to follow the journey of self discovery and to look at life through fresh eyes. Take time to smell the roses, view the sunsets and sunrises, look at the moon differently, look at people's smiles, their words, and thoughts more intensely. Make a difference in people's lives by touching them with your strength, courage and self confidence.

Remember to bring out the best in other people by praising others liberally, listening to them and helping them. People come in all sizes, shapes, colors, and flavors. They come from all walks of life and have much to offer. People are what makes this world the world it is today. Our lives are enriched by people, some more valuable, some more gentle, but all have gifts. At the ends of your days, you want to think back, I've been blessed by who I have known, whose lives I have touched, and what I have learned from others.

Family Physician:

1.How often should I have a mammogram?

2.How often should I have a clinical breast exam?

3.How often should I do a breast self exam?

4.Do you want to know my family history of breast cancer as well as other cancers?

5.What other tests do you recommend for high risk women?

6.What do BIRAD scores stand for?

7. How do they measure breast density on a mammogram and ultrasound?

8.Do I have dense breasts?

Breast Center:

1.How often should I have a mammogram and clinical breast exam?

2.How often should I do a breast self exam?

3.What time of the month should I do a breast self exam?

4.Do you want to write down my family history of breast cancer and cancer?

5.Do I have dense breasts?

6. What is my BIRAD score?

Radiologist:

1.Are there any other tests you'd recommend for my breast cancer diagnosis? (That is if you have a hereditary cancer in your family, you are from a high risk family history with relatives who have had breast cancer, or in a high risk age category?)

2.What type of biopsy will you be doing? Please explain the procedure to me.

3.When will I get the results? Can I get a written copy of the report as well?

4.How soon after the biopsy can I shower or take a bath? When can I take the bandage off?

Breast Cancer Nurse Practitioner:

Before Surgery:

1.What is the name of my type of cancer? What is the stage? What is the grade?

2.Can you explain the pathology report to me in more detail?

3.What are my treatment options?

4.How much time do I have to consider the treatment options?

5.What do you feel is my prognosis?

6.What happens when the surgeon does a lumpectomy? What will I look like? What are the chances of a reccurrence ?

7.What happens when the surgeon does a mastectomy? What will I look like? What are the chances of a reccurrence?

8.What would you do?

9.Would you recommend going to a breast cancer support group, seeing a therapist, counselor or social worker?

After Surgery:

1. How large was the tumor? Was the tumor in the ducts (in situ) or invasive (grown through the ducts)?
2. What stage of cancer do I have? What grade do I have?
3. Please explain the stages and grades to me.
4. Would you explain the updated pathology report to me?
5. What are my treatment options?
6. How much time do I have to consider the options?
7. What treatments would you do with this prognosis?
8. What is the significance of cancer spreading to my lymph nodes?
9. Was my tumor checked for estrogen and progesterone by a receptor test? What do the results positive and negative mean?
10. Please exam the Her2/neu test to me.
11. Please explain the fish test to me.

Breast Surgeon:

Before Surgery:

1. What experience do you have in treating breast cancer? Do you do breast surgery often?
2. What type of surgery are you recommending for me? Is this the least invasive procedure and safest?
3. What are the advantages and disadvantages of a lumpectomy? What is the chance of reccurrence?
4. What type of incision will you be doing? Lumpectomy? Segmental incision? Tylectomy incision?
5. What are the types of mastectomies? What are the advantages and disadvantages of a mastectomy? What are the chances of reccurrence?
6. How long will I be in the hospital?
7. What's a sentinel node biopsy? Axillary dissection?
8. Should I see a genetic counselor?
9. Should other female family members in my family be screened for breast cancer?
10. Will I have the same ability to enjoy sex after breast cancer surgery?

After Surgery:

1. How large was my tumor?
2. What stage is it?
3. What grade is it?
4. What is the name of my type of cancer?
5. How many lymph nodes were removed?
6. What size were they?
7. Was the sentinelnode removed?
8. In which level of the axillary gland were the nodes removed?
9. Will I get lymphedema or swelling in my arm? How can I prevent lymph edema?
10. When will the drain under my arm be removed?

11. What exercises should I do after surgery? When should I start them?

12. Do you expect the tumor to have invaded the breast or arm tissue?

13. How long will I be in the hospital?

14. When will the stitches be removed? When do I come back?

15. What is the chance of reccurrence in this breast? The other breast?

16. Do you think I will need radiation, chemo, hormone therapy?

17. Will I need physical therapy?

18. What physical activities am I allowed to do after surgery?

16. What can I do for pain?

17. When do I come back for a check up on my surgical site and drain? What is the follow up care?

18. How long before I can do housework, return to work, or resume my daily leisure activities?

19. Should I see a genetic counselor? (Tell me the reasons why you think I should.)

20. Should my female family members be screened for breast cancer?

21. Will having breast cancer surgery effect the feelings in my breast, the ability to enjoy sex?

Reconstructive Surgeon:

1. Should I have immediate reconstruction at the time of the surgery? Should the surgery be delayed? How long?

1. What will I look like if I have plastic surgery?

2. What is the difference between a tram flap, lattimus flap, and implant? What are the advantages and disadvantages of each?

3. What surgery would you recommend for me?

4. Could you show me pictures of each of these procedures?

5. How many years do the flaps and implants last? What are the complications from each of them?

6. What are the risks of capsular contracture?

7. Are there any books or videos you recommend that I watch?

Mastectomy Shop:

1. What prostheses are available? What are the advantages and disadvantages of all of these?

2. What items do you have for lymphedema, in case I get it?

Oncologist:

1. What is my diagnosis? Tell me what staging is? What is my tumor grade? What is my cancer type?

2. Can I get a copy of my results?

3. What are my treatment options? What are the benefits and side effects from each treatment? (short term and long term) Do you recommend a second opinion?

4. What are the clinical trials available in which I would qualify for? What are the

pros and cons of each? Risk factors for each? How is this different from the standard treatment? Will my drugs or treatment be paid for? What are the risks from being in a clinical trial? Will my health care be the same?

5.What effect will my treatment have on menopause, my sex life, pregnancy, and being able to breast feed?

6.Are phytoestrogens (plant estrogens) good for me to take if I'm estrogen positive?

7.How does my family history of breast , ovarian, endometrial cancer effect treatment choices?

8.How does a strong family history of breast cancer effect my treatment choices?

Hormone Therapy:

1.What hormone drugs do you recommend? What are the side effects of the various drugs? What are the long term risks from the various drugs? Which hormone therapy has the highest risk of side effects? What can I do to reduce my risk of long term side effects?

Chemotherapy:

1.Do I need chemotherapy? What is my cancer stage and how does this determine the types of treatment necessary?

2.What chemo drugs will I be given? What are the short term side effects? The long term side effects?

3.How many months will the treatments last?

4.How will the chemo be given? IV, oral pills, or both?

5.Will I be given anti nausea pills? How often will I need to take them?

6.What are the side effects from this treatment?

7.What is a port?

8.Will I be able to use birth control pills?

9.What are the restrictions on activities and eating while going through chemo treatments?

10.What are the chances that my tumor will not respond to chemo?

11.Who do I call if I have side effects?

12. When are the side effects serious enough to be hospitalized?

13.What effect will chemo have on future pregnancies, menstruation, and getting cancer again? Will I go into early menopause? Will I be able to breast feed? Will this effect my sex life?

14.What are the signs of metastasis?

15.How does my family history of breast, ovarian, endometrial cancer effect my treatment choices? How does a strong family history of breast cancer effect my treatment options?

Radiation Oncologist:

1. How many treatments will I receive? How long are the treatments? Where will I receive the treatments?

2.How long will be my first treatment be to mark the areas?

3.What are the long term and short term effects from this treatment?

4.What is my risk of recurrence?

5.What side effects should I call you about immediately?

6.What are the bathing and showering recommendations?

7.Is there anything I can use on the treatment area during this time period?

8.Can I shave and use deodorant under my arm? Should I wear a bra?

9.Can I use sunscreen when I go outside?

10.What should I eat while going through radiation treatments?

11.Should all my dental work be done before radiation?

American Cancer Society
1-800-ACS-2345 (National Office) www.cancer.org

American Institute of Cancer Research
1-800-843-8114

Avon Breast Cancer Crusade
www.avoncrusade.com
An organization that funds access to care and wants to find a cure for breast cancer
through fund raising activities and products.

The Breast Cancer Fund
1-415-346-8223 www.breastcancerfund.org

Breastcancer.org
www.breastcancer.org
A nonprofit website that is dedicated to providing the most reliable and complete
information available.

Cancer Care
1-800-813-HOPE www.cancercare.org

Cancercervive
1-800-486-2874 www.cancervive.org

Cancer Hope Network
1-877-HOPENET www.cancerhopenetwork.org

Cancer Information Hotline
1-800-525-3777

Cancer Information Service (CIS)
1-800-4-CANCER www.nci.nih.gov

Cancer Wellness Center
1-847-509-9494 www.cancedrwellness.org

Celebrating Life Foundation (CIF)
1-800-207-0992 www.celebratinglife.org
A nonprofit organization devoted to educating women of color.

Inflammatory Breast Cancer Research Foundation
877-786-7422 www.ibcresearch.org
This site provides education, active participation in research and links to clinical information.

Living Beyond Breast Cancer
800-753-5222 www.lbbc.org
This site provides educational materials, a quarterly newsletter, and a Young Survivors network.

Men Against Breast Cancer
866-547-6222 www.menagainstbreastcancer.org
This site mobilizes men to fight to eradicate of breast cancer and support men whose families are going through breast cancer.

National Alliance of Breast Cancer Organizations (NABCO)
1-800-719-9154 www.nabco.org

National Breast Cancer Organization
1-800-221-2141

National Coalition for Cancer Survivorship
1-888-YES-NCCS www.cansearch.org

National Lymphedema Network
1-800-541-3259 www.lymphnet.org
A nonprofit organization that provides guidance and educational materials to patients.

Sisters Network, Inc.
866-781-1808 www.sisternetworkin.org
An organization that seeks to increase attention to the impact breast cancer has in the African American community.

Susan G. Komen Breast Cancer Foundation
800-462-9273 www.komen.org
This is a toll-free breast cancer helpline where you can discuss your breast cancer problems. There is breast cancer materials available.

Y-ME National Breast Cancer Organization, Inc.
800-221-2141(English) or 800-986-9505(Spanish) www.y-me.org
They have a hotline to discuss breast cancer with women and their families.

Young Survival Coalition
212-916-7667 www.youngsurvival.org
An organization dedicated to the breast cancer issues of women under 40 years of age.

YWCA Encore Plus Program
1-800-95E PLUS www.ywca.org/html/B4d1.asp

Breast Cancer happens to nice people and often for no rhyme or reason. You may have been chosen, so turn it around and do some good for others by touching their lives. Be a volunteer or spokesperson in your community.

Review your goals and purpose in life. Do you have your priorities in order? Do you have a balance in your home life? Workplace? Within your body? Do you eat nutritionally? Do you monitor the stressors in your life? Do you watch the toxins in your environment? Do you have spiritual faith?

Exercise your body, as it's the machine that sets the stage for cancer. Our society is confronted with too many people with health problems. These problems are caused by poor diet, lack of exercise, daily stressors and environmental toxicity.

Accept your prognosis of cancer and find the cause by working vigilantly with your team of qualified medical doctors. Determine from this experience what's important and what's not. Don't let the emotional scars and cosmetic disability stay with you. It's what's inside that counts.

Stress can cause a lot of imbalance in your body, so it's important to find ways to release and balance the stressors in your life. Activities like meditation, counseling, yoga, and a strong network of friends help to release stress. Laugh often, have a lot of hope, keep a positive attitude, and be flexible.

Treatment is important to your care. Early diagnosis is of utmost importance. Work with your medical team to have a well balanced treatment for the whole person--physiological, psychological and nutritionally.

Cancer is a wake up call. Look for the signs you may have missed. Care about yourself and even those who don't understand cancer. You can be a light in the darkness.

Answer to God and trust in the plan He has for you. Do you have strong faith in a supreme being? Your life is in his hands and it's up to your grace to fulfill it. Have faith in today, tomorrow and the future.

Networks of support are important to everyone. Search out others who are in need. Make a difference in the world by giving of yourself.

Count your many blessings and share them with others. If you can teach, teach. If you can speak, speak. If you can do, do. If you can make, make. If you can share, share.

Express your feelings, don't keep them bottled up inside. Get rid of the reasons for health problems. Breathe in good stressors and exhale bad stresses.

Rejoice in life, cherish and be grateful for each and every moment. Live normally. Value the time you have on earth by celebrating life.

"Peggy" Margaret A. Anderson is a retired teacher from Duluth Public Schools. Peggy retired in 2003 after 28 years of teaching in ISD 709. In Duluth schools she taught all grades in one way or another, including special education. As a goal setter, she aimed to teach all grades to understand the whole learning development pattern of students. She could be termed as a "professional student." Peggy graduated from Bemidji State University in 1971, got her master's degree from the University of Minnesota in 1987. While going to college and teaching, Peggy obtained eight teaching licensures, one being an administrative license. She took many credits in art and physical education in college as well. After retiring, Peggy went back to college to work on her doctorate in education before being faced with a different challenge. She hopes to go back in the next year, and also continue her drawing classes.

The schools she taught at in Duluth Public Schools include: Washington Junior, West Junior, Park Point Elementary, Lester Park Elementary, Chester Park Elementary, Ordean Junior High and Central High School. She has been involved in numerous summer school programs including teaching writing at Ordean, Park Point and Woodland Hills programs. In her teaching career she taught in St. Peter Public Schools, was a summer coordinator in St. Peter Public Schools, was assistant director and teacher of Northland Day Activity Center International Falls, and long term substitute teacher in Littlefork, Loman, and International Falls school systems.

Peggy completed her Master's degree in 1987. The thesis topic was "Individualized Testing and Specific Reading Games and Activities That Could Enhance Reading Development in First Grade." Her advisor, Dr. Helen Carlson had her complete it in a book format. She strove to teach students who were struggling with reading by a multisensory approach to reading. Peggy was a speaker at ADK on genealogy with the topic being Tracing Your Family Tree. She and her husband, Jim, were speakers at The Minnesota Council for the Gifted and Talented in 1990. Their presentation was Thinking, Writing, and Literature Activities-a Potpourri of Ideas to Bring Back to Your Classroom. She was involved in writing other curriculum as well.

Peg's greatest honors were being nominated for Minnesota Teacher of the Year (1990) and the Ashland Individual Teacher Award (1989). She was always a teacher who strove for excellence and this was displayed in her graduate credits with a 3.9 GPA.

In the public and private school systems, Peggy is known in many circles. In the Duluth schools she belonged to the school district System Accountability committee, special ed committees, OBE, SST, representative positions, and site team committees. In the schools she was involved with the gifted program. Peggy was an Odyssey of the Mind coach and coordinator at Chester Park and at Holy Rosary as well as OM judge. She was involved with Holy Rosary, Marshall, East, Lester Park, and Chester Park's PTA's.

At UMD, she is known for being a member of the Teacher Education Council as well as supervising student teachers from UMD and St. Scholastica, and member of Phi Delta Kappa. She was a member of Phi Kappa Pi as well.

In the community, Peggy is presently involved as heart volunteer each year, belongs to four luncheon groups, is a member of the Spirit Team Board, is an advocate for the American Cancer Society, is a member of Faith investment club and is involved in many numerous activities. She was a member of the Duluth Playhouse, co-leader of the Lester Park Dinosaur Club, Lester Park Hockey Association, the Duluth Women's Club, the Arrowhead Reading Association, Minnesota Reading Association, International Reading Association, Council for the Gifted, Kappa Delta Pi, Early Childhood Association, Boy Scout merit badge counselor and Alpha Delta Kappa board member. She has been involved in community ed and art classes through the years. Peggy is a former member of Lutheran Church of Good Shepherd where she and her husband were co-superintendents of Sunday school for several years and taught grief classes. They are very involved at Faith Lutheran Church presently. She enjoys giving to organizations and making gifts for individuals.

Outside of Duluth, Peggy, was involved in being a Brownie and Girl Scout leader, ARC, CEC organizations and on the board of Minnie Ahmik along with many educational activities.

A picture of Peggy with her daughter, Lisa, at the Mother's Day Walk Run in Duluth, MN wearing their home-made lumpectomy tie dyed T-shirts.

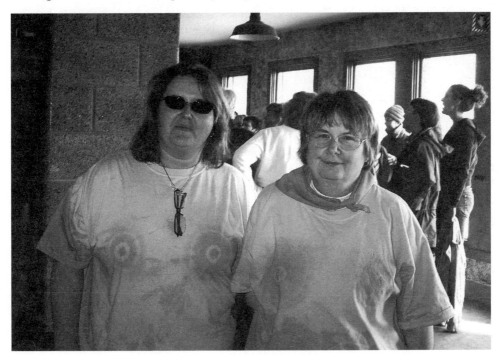

Chemo Cocktail Resource Guide

Typical Common Chemo Drugs That Can Be Used In Any Combination:
1.CMF-cytoxan or cyclophosphamide, methotrexate, 5-FU or 5 flurorouracil
2.CAF-adriamycin or doxorubicin, cyclophosphamide, 5 fluorouracil
3.CFP-prednisone, 5-FU, cytoxan
4.CMFVP-cytoxan, methrotrexate, 5-FU, viscristine, prednisone
5.FAC-adriamycin, cytoxan, 5-FU
6.Other drugs could include: CEF, CMFVP, AC, VAT, VATH, CDDP ,and VP-16 plus VP-16, AC plus T, AC plus Txt

The Most Common Drugs Fall Into These Categories:

1.Antibotics-These are used to stop DNA from replicating. Examples could include doxorubicin or Adriamycin (A) and epirubicin (E) or Ellence.
2.Alkylators-Drugs that stop cell division and growth. Examples cyclophosphamide or Cytoxan-C
3.Antimetabolities-These are drugs that cause the cells to die and prevent them from dividing as well. Examples of these drugs are Methotrexate, 5-fluorouracil, capecitabine or Xeloda, and gemcitabine or Gemzar.
4.Antimicrotubles-Drugs that kill the cancer cells and spare the normal cells. Examples can include Taxanes as paclitaxel or Taxol, docetaxel or Taxotere, vincristine or Oncovin, vinblastine or Velban, and vinorelbine or Navelbine.

How Are Chemo Drugs Given?

Chemo drugs are given several ways: 1.by mouth 2.muscle injections 3.injections into fatty body tissues and by 4.IV's.

To purchase copies of, *Dear Auntie, Why Me?*

(This is a true story of a Duluth woman's struggle with breast cancer. It includes letters to her Auntie and replies as well as numerous illustrations, charts, pictures, positive affirmations they shared, and is jam packed full of information on breast cancer that she wished she would of known before a diagnosis of breast cancer.)

Write this e-mail address: kc0mko@charter.net
                     e-mail address: maande1@charter.net
Address: Peggy Anderson Publishing
             5204 Otsego St.
             Duluth, MN 55804
Or call: 218-525-1905
Fax: 218-525-3539
Toll free: 1-800-900-4559 (00)
Cost: $21.44 (with taxes)-check or money order
Shipping: This applies to out of the Duluth area orders. For uninsured, book rate please allow $5.00 extra dollars. I will send you a check back with the book if there's a left over balance. If it's more, I will bill you.
Proceeds: The proceeds of this book are being donated to SMDC foundation for breast cancer training, and diagnostic and treatment machines, after taxes are paid.

Name:_____

Address:_____

City, State, Zip Code:_____

Phone number_____

Thank you!!!! Thank you!!!!!

(Bookstore vendors: reseller discounts are available.)